Chronic Pain:
America's Hidden Epidemic

CHRONIC PAIN:

America's Hidden Epidemic

EDITED BY
Steven F. Brena, M.D.

ATHENEUM/SMI *New York* 1978

TO THE INJURED WORKER,
one of the countless victims of learned pain.

Library of Congress Cataloging in Publication Data

Main entry under title:
Chronic pain.
Bibliography: p.
Includes index.
1. Pain. I. Brena, Steven F. [DNLM:
1. Pain. 2. Chronic disease. WL704 C557]
RB127.C48 616'.047 77-15888
ISBN 0-689-10874-5

Published simultaneously in Canada by McClelland and Stewart Ltd.
Manufactured by American Book-Stratford Press, Saddle Brook, New Jersey
Designed by Kathleen Carey
First Edition

Introduction

PAIN IS ONE OF the most important concerns of humankind and a factor that has influenced history. This is documented in the records of every race and civilization: in the cave drawings of prehistoric man, in the oldest written documents of ancient China, on Babylonian clay tablets and papyri written in the days of the pyramid builders, on Persian leather documents, and on the parchment scrolls from Troy.

Through the ages we see ubiquitous testimonials to the omnipresence of pain. "Were we to imagine ourselves," wrote the French surgeon Louis Dartigues, "suspended in timeless space over an abyss of which the sounds of revolving earth rose to our ears, we would hear naught but an elemental roar of pain uttered as with one voice by suffering mankind."

While acute pain serves a useful purpose—it warns us when something is wrong and helps the physician make a diagnosis—pain in its chronic form is a malefic force which imposes severe emotional, physical, economic, and sociologic stresses on the patient, the family, and society. As John Milton so elegantly stated in *Paradise Lost,* Book VI:

> But pain is perfect miserie, the worst
> Of evils, and excessive, overturns
> All patience . . .

Because chronic pain is the most frequent cause of disability, it constitutes a major national and world health and economic problem. Although accurate statistics are not available, data from a variety of sources suggest that chronic-pain states cost the American people between $40 and $50 billion annually for hospital, medical, and other health services and from loss of work productivity.

Even more important is the cost in terms of human suffering. It is a distressing fact that, in this age of marvelous scientific and technological advances that permit us to send people to the moon, there are millions of suffering patients who are not getting relief. Many of these patients are exposed to a high risk of medically induced complications from improper therapy, including narcotic addiction, or receive multiple, often useless, and at times mutilating operations. A significant number give up medical care and consult quacks who not only deplete the patient's financial resources but often do harm; some patients with severe, intractable pain become so desperate as to commit suicide.

The many reasons for the less-than-optimal care of patients with chronic pain can be grouped into three major categories: voids in our knowledge, improper application of the knowledge we have available, and inadequate communication between patient and physician and among physicians and scientists.

Even though we've accumulated a great deal of knowledge about *acute* pain in the century and a half since the scientific study of pain began, this knowledge has not been very useful to *chronic*-pain patients because of the difference between acute and chronic pain. Moreover, while medical students, physicians, and health professionals are learning how to manage acute pain, few, if any, schools teach the basic principles essential to making a correct diagnosis and formulating the proper therapy for patients with chronic pain.

Although a few pioneers long ago emphasized the marked difference between acute and chronic pain, this was ignored until recently, and physicians treated patients with chronic pain the same as those with acute pain. A related factor is the progressive trend toward specialization, in which each specialist views pain in a narrow, "tubular" fashion according to his or her own specialty. Finally, there is the problem of inadequate or total lack of communication among the variety of people involved in this problem.

The public has continued to accept pain as one of the natural consequences of disease. This, together with the fact that physicians and other health professionals have not fully appreciated or even realized the magnitude of this serious disease state, has resulted in totally inadequate scientific research and teaching programs and relative neglect of the unfortunate chronic sufferers.

Fortunately, during the past decade or so several changes have taken place which, if they grow and continue, promise to assist our health professions in coping with this problem. For one thing, there is a move by scientists and clinicians to collaborate in studying the basic mechanisms and the physical and behavioral characteristics of chronic-pain syndromes—an essential step toward proper diagnosis and therapy of such problems. Animal models have been developed in an attempt toward clarifying the basic disorders of nerves, muscles, and organs that help produce chronic pain. In addition to obtaining new information relevant to chronic pain, collaboration between scientists and clinicians will result in more rapid application of this new knowledge to the treatment of patients.

Another important advance has been the recent surge of interest in the organization and operation of multidisciplinary pain-treatment or pain-rehabilitation centers or clinics. Such facilities usually include a number of health professionals from different disciplines who work as a coordinated team. Each member of the team has special interests, knowledge, and skills in managing patients with chronic pain and is willing to pool his talents with those of other members. The common goal is to make a correct diagnosis and develop plans for the best therapy for each patient.

This book is a good example of the kind of well-coordinated team effort that is significantly improving the care of patients with chronic pain. Dr. Brena has been my friend for a quarter of a century and was a close associate and collaborator for a number of years. He has used his vast knowledge and broad experience in the field of pain therapy in developing a comprehensive format for the book, including in it some of the most important and interesting aspects of pain.

Under his leadership, each contributor—an authority in his or her discipline—has done an admirable job of evaluating, distilling, and interpreting a vast amount of scientific information and presenting it in a lucid and easily readable form. Therefore, the book will have a special appeal to the general reader and should be extremely useful to victims of chronic pain and their families, relatives, and friends.

The fact that the book limits the use of scientific or medical "jargon" should prove a refreshing change from the traditionally ponderous format and language of medical articles and textbooks. In addition, the book should prove especially informative and useful to practitioners who have not had ample opportunities to gain experience in the management of patients with chronic pain. It will acquaint them with the "behavioral model" of pain introduced a few years ago, along with therapeutic options that are now available as a result of this concept.

Finally, it is hoped that the book will help the American people better appreciate the importance of chronic pain as a major national health and economic problem. Hopefully, this will encourage them to support the multipronged attack essential to its solution: greater research efforts, expanded clinical facilities, and better teaching programs—all leading to better care of chronic-pain patients. While the attack on chronic pain must be made by scientists and health professionals, public support and greatly increased funds and resources will be necessary if we are to mount a massive "crash" program such as we have launched against cancer, heart disease, and other serious health problems. Only in this way will suffering humanity obtain relief.

John J. Bonica, M.D., D.Sc.

Contents

PART II CHRONIC PAIN AND THE INDIVIDUAL

Contributors

(IN ALPHABETICAL ORDER)

WILLIAM H. BIGGERS, M.D. *Professor of Psychiatry, Emory University School of Medicine*

JOHN J. BONICA, M.D. *President, International Association for Study on Pain; Professor of Anesthesiology, University of Washington School of Medicine, Seattle, Washington*

VERNON L. BRECKNER, M.D. *Professor of Anesthesiology; Director, Pain Manage-*

ment Clinic; University of California at Los Angeles School of Medicine

STEVEN F. BRENA, M.D. — *Associate Professor of Anesthesiology and Rehabilitation Medicine; Director, Pain Control Center; Emory University School of Medicine*

STANLEY L. CHAPMAN, PH.D. — *Instructor in Psychology, Department of Rehabilitation Medicine; Staff Member, Emory Pain Control Center; Emory University School of Medicine*

SAMUEL B. CHYATTE, M.D. — *Professor of Rehabilitation Medicine; Director, Disability Clinic and Teaching and Research Center; Emory University School of Medicine*

ROBIN J. DE ANDRADE, M.D. — *Professor of Rehabilitation Medicine and Orthopedic Surgery; Chairman, Department of Rehabilitation Medicine; Emory University School of Medicine*

THERESA FERRER-BRECKNER, M.D. — *Associate Professor of Anesthesiology, Pain Management Clinic; University of California at Los Angeles School of Medicine*

WILLIAM D. HAMMONDS, M.D. — *Assistant Professor of Anesthesiology and Rehabilitation Medicine; Staff Member, Emory Pain Control Center; Emory University School of Medicine*

EDWARD E. SAMMONS, M.D. — *Assistant Professor of Anesthesiology and Rehabilitation Medicine; Staff Member, Emory Pain Control Center; Emory University School of Medicine*

NORMAN C. SHEALY, M.D., PH.D. — *Director, Pain and Health Rehabilitation Center,® La Crosse, Wisconsin*

IRVING P. UNIKEL, PH.D. — *Professor in Psychology, Department of Psychiatry; Senior Consultant, Emory Pain Control Center; Emory University School of Medicine*

PART I

Chronic Pain and the American Society

EDITOR'S NOTE: *The term "American Society" is used here according to Toynbee's definition. It doesn't mean the "American people," but the network of relationships among Americans.*

1

The Staggering Cost of Chronic Pain

S. F. BRENA

ABOUT ONE MILLION American workers on any given day are crippled by chronic pain. At an average cost in medical care of $40 per individual, the bill in 1974 came to $14.6 billion. This figure does not take into account the billions of dollars lost in man-days of work, compensation payments, and litigation costs.

In 1973, the people of California paid something like $200 million for chronic low back pain alone.

For the year 1976, the Georgia Board of Workmen's Compensation shows a bill of $38,392,911 for medical and compensation payments, with 1,941,058 lost days of work. Of these cases, over one third involved minor accidents, such as sprains and strains, where the only disabling factor was pain.

The National Institute of Arthritis research estimates that about 21 million Americans are affected by arthritis. Most of them are disabled by pain and not by damage to bodily function due to the arthritis process, with an estimated cost of $11 billion for medical care and 200 million work-days lost.

Data quoted by John Bonica indicate that about 25 million Americans are suffering from recurrent headaches with a loss of about 180 million work-days and a total cost of about $10 billion. Many of the patients seen at the University of Washington Pain Center in Seattle, directed by Dr. Bonica, have paid over $40,000 in health care; the cost of the most complex pain problems, together with the loss of work productivity, amounts to over $125,000 per patient. And these figures do not reflect the enormous social wreckage in terms of drug misuse, depression, and wasted lives.

Chronic pain is a staggering social and economic problem, almost totally ignored by the American public and a majority of health professionals. The lack of a constructive policy in dealing with chronic pain has caused billions of dollars to be drained from the U.S. Treasury in Social Security disability payments to chronic-pain sufferers, other billions to be paid by insurance firms to pain patients, egged on by "whiplash lawyers" who sue for injury and malpractice. Tragically, many of the legal steps we take to protect the individual sufferer and to increase his or her chance for health have worked instead to perpetuate the misery of learned helplessness and depression in millions of people.

The epidemic of chronic disabling pain in our society has magnified a strictly medical problem into a major social issue. Just as pain in the individual is a warning that something is wrong either physically or emotionally—

quite often both—the "pain epidemic" can be viewed as an alarm signaling to us that something is wrong with our social philosophy and laws.

Two distinct types of pain—acute and chronic—are commonly seen by doctors. Acute pain is usually associated with a specific disease or injury. If you burn your hand on a hot coffee-pot, the feeling you get is one of acute pain; it can be traced to a stimulus (the hot coffee-pot), and the pain will often disappear shortly after the stimulus is removed, when the pot is dropped or placed on a table.

It is chronic pain that presents an enigma. Chronic pain lingers far beyond the time when a simple cause-and-effect relationship might have explained the problem, and many physicians are baffled when they try to find the origins of a patient's chronic suffering. Although chronic pain is usually triggered by an injury or disease, it is continued indefinitely by a multitude of factors, including ethnic and cultural influences, emotional reactions, and secondary gains or pay-offs from chronic-pain behavior.

Why this particular problem today? Several factors have contributed to making chronic pain a major problem of the twentieth century, whereas in earlier times it was not nearly so prevalent.

First: Paradoxically, the triumph of science in controlling infectious diseases and in saving lives after severe injury has upset the Darwinian principle of "survival of the fittest." From an ecological view, modern medicine is one of the earth's greatest pollutants, keeping alive, but unproductive, individuals who otherwise would be long dead.

This prolongation of human life has created enormous social and medical problems, most of which are connected with the aging process. Chronic degenerative diseases, largely age-related, have replaced infectious diseases as one of the leading causes of illness among Americans. Many degenerative changes, especially those in the spine and weight-bearing joints, are painful and may be disabling enough to carry a related emotional impact.

Second: If medicine has upset the laws of survival, it has also failed to help those whose lives were saved, so that they might enjoy their new lease on life. Millions of patients have gone through extensive surgical procedures requiring weeks of inactivity, total dependence, and heavy drug intake. On discharge, these patients often continue their learned sick-and-drug behavior without being properly re-educated. Society will pay such people for being sick. It is not yet ready to deal with them in more positive ways.

Looking back a little over a century, the soldiers of Abraham Lincoln and Jefferson Davis died by the scores of thousands from battle wounds and disease; thousands more died who would have been saved had there been modern emergency medical care. But those who lasted knew they had to pull themselves together quickly. They knew that to continue surviving they had to return to productivity in a society that had not yet invented welfare programs and the Veterans Administration.

Third: Over the past thirty years, the medical profession and related agencies that promote health have conducted intensive educational campaigns to acquaint the public with disease symptoms. Today, terms such as angina pectoris, arthritis, hypertension, leukemia, and multiple sclerosis are practically household words.

This emphasis on sickness-awareness may be useful in alerting people against diseases. It may have helped in the prevention and early treatment of potentially deadly disorders such as high blood-pressure and cancer. At the same time, though, sickness-awareness has created a tremendous disease-phobia; one example is the widespread compulsive fear of having cancer.

From media information on illness, we have vicariously picked up symptoms of diseases that most of us formerly would not have heard about. We behave like the medical student who begins to detect in himself the signs of an illness he or she reads about in medical textbooks. Many people crowd the offices of physicians and hospital emergency rooms with a variety of complaints that express nothing more than a neurotic fear of having heart disease, cancer, and other mysterious disorders. Sick behaviors are being reinforced by those very institutions that are supposed to help in restoring health.

If, on a tour of Europe, you had an opportunity to visit an early hospital such as the famous Hôtel des Dieux in Paris, you would be surprised by the horrors that sufferers of earlier times endured. People were jammed together in large wards of 50–100 beds, with no privacy, no personal-hygiene facilities, no certified nurses, and of course, none of the present-day amenities such as TVs and lounges. These were places where people went for treatment, and they looked forward to getting out as quickly as possible.

Compare those institutions with our modern hospitals, which compete with each other to provide deluxe services just as hotels and motels do. Today's highly trained nurses tend to pamper the hospital's clientele into a feeling of total dependence. Think of the businesses that have grown up around hospitals: the get-well cards, the bouquets of flowers, the social entertaining that occurs in the rooms of sick people. We are not advocating a return to cruder hospital facilities as a means of eradicating learned pain and sickness; we are only pointing out why the sick role is often pleasant enough to continue indefinitely in people who are prone to develop learned pain behaviors.

Fourth: Accidents rank third after heart disease and cancer as the leading cause of death among Americans today. Those who survive are often left crippled for life in a hopeless situation of learned pain; many unnecessarily swell the files of those prematurely retired on Social Security benefits. Some people who've suffered a whiplash contusion in a car accident adopt a permanent lifestyle of misery and drugs, with no real evidence of anatomical damage, but with a great deal of pressure on them to maintain their sick behavior.

Accidents are frequently linked to the epidemic abuse of drugs for emotional needs. The law recognizes alcohol intoxication as one of the leading causes of traffic accidents. But why not address the dangers of driving under the influence of tranquilizers, opiates, and amphetamines (the pep-drugs)? How many workers clumsily hurt themselves on the job for the same reason?

Files at the Emory University Pain Control Center in Atlanta document repeated accidents among people who habitually misuse drugs. A common example is that of John B., who was released after being treated in a hospital for an acute injury. He returned to work without first being detoxified of the drugs he had been given, and a few weeks later was involved in a car accident. John was hurt again and disabled indefinitely, because his performance had been impaired by Valium, codeine, and other drugs that affected his motor coordination and judgment.

Chronic pain is a recognizable disease state involving many factors that interact with one another. Among the peculiarities of chronic pain is the way it is reinforced by its own consequences rather than being dependent on any given physical insult or damage to the body. We commonly see five consequences in chronic pain—known among pain experts as the "Five D's" syndrome:

1. *Drug Misuse.* People in pain usually take painkillers. Many kill themselves slowly by drug intoxication while receiving little pain relief.

2. *Dysfunction.* People in pain often decrease their activities, their range of joint-motion, and change their ways of walking, sitting, and standing. Each of these reductions in performance is likely to produce strains and distortions in different groups of muscles, causing greater discomfort.

3. *Disuse.* When dysfunction reaches levels of near or total inactivity of certain groups of muscles or of the whole body, various painful organic lesions develop. Common examples of "disuse" lesions are the so-called frozen or stiff joints and osteoporosis, a dangerous softening of the bone that causes the individual to have a high risk of fractures.

4. *Depression.* People in pain are depressed; this is often a consequence of not being able to do what they formerly did and enjoyed. People in pain have lost the "flavor" of life; they have become hopelessly dependent upon others for their needs. In turn, depression makes people more "pain-prone." If there is a dog barking outside your window and you are doing things you like to do, you will scarcely notice the noise. The dog's barking is always the same; it is your state of mind and activity that condition your sensory experience. When some people quit being active and start "listening" compulsively to their bodily "barks," their pain has a tendency to increase to intolerable levels.

5. *Disability.* People with pain, dysfunction, and

disuse often lose the ability to perform their jobs. For this they receive compensation from our compassionate American culture. While such compensation may be ethically justified and socially and legally approved, we can see on every hand that a long-term disability income triggers a state of learned helplessness. The habit of relying on others for an income slowly destroys our confidence in ourselves, decreases our willingness to keep active and productive, depresses our emotional drives, and increases our dysfunction, disuse, and drug problems, ultimately leading to almost unbearable suffering.

2

Why Man Alone Has Chronic Pain

S. F. BRENA

THERE IS NOT MUCH difference between the pain response of a wounded lion in America and a wounded lion in Africa, but there are enormous differences in human pain-behaviors even when sufferers belong to the same cultural group.

Man suffers in a different way and possibly much more than the animal because man alone among all living creatures is self-conscious. He is aware of himself as different from others, with a unique personality that belongs to him alone. When injury or disease strikes, it is not simply the affected limb or inner organ that hurts; man's entire personality is called into the experience and is affected and sometimes damaged in the process.

There are times when pain has great value. Nature devised pain as a warning signal when some bodily function or organ has been threatened. Indeed, the fact that pain is everywhere is a testimonial to its worth as a survival mechanism. Nature did not intend that pain should be a *chronic* source of distress, however. Only man seems capable of this kind of irrational behavior, helped along, ironically, by his superior intellect and by the environmental systems he has designed for better living conditions.

All animals are highly efficient in the skills that allow them to survive. When confronted by danger, the antelope can outrun most pursuers, the elephant has greater physical strength, and the chameleon can fool the smartest predator with its camouflage skills. Even though the nervous system of an animal may be relatively primitive, increasing in complexity as it moves up the evolutionary scale, each animal system does provide a means by which its owner can escape or overcome its enemies.

The nervous structures of animals are best designed to provide expression of the "instinct," a built-in, fixed species-behavior, with few and minor individual variations. The animal does not need to "think" in order to survive: Nature has provided it, through its own species, with a survival blueprint that leaves it little freedom of choice. Acting by reflex, animals do not need an elaborate nervous system to defend against environmental, body-damaging threats.

Pound for pound of body weight, man is one of the weakest of all creatures. His survival skill rests instead on his intelligence, on his power of independent, imaginative thinking. From the Stone Age to the present, man has outsmarted, outrun, outfought, and dominated all other living creatures by using his intellectual skills. We can see this brain power in the many tools he has invented to compensate for his lack of both great physical strength and in-born instinct. Man has no instinct to rely on in the face of challenge. The so-called human instincts actually are learned habits that must be cultivated and exercised in order to be useful.

The evolutionary process has granted man a newer, more sophisticated nervous system capable of swiftly relaying to the brain messages concerning threats to the well-being of the body. Our responses to the pain experience are never merely nervous reflexes, as in animals, but always, even in the most acute emergencies, the ultimate expression of an intricate, integrated brain process involving both cognitive and emotional factors.

If your hand is burned by a hot coffee-pot, you are not likely to simply drop the pot to avoid further damage; rather, you will evaluate your damage as it relates to your environment and to memories of past experiences. You may drop the pot if you are in a campground, but you are likely to hold it a little longer in order to safely deposit it on a table if the mishap occurs while you are standing on a rich Oriental rug in the home of your boss. In doing so, you have exercised an intelligent choice, one which is not a mere reflex.

Initially, pain can have a very useful function, because it triggers a corrective action directed mainly toward the quenching of the acute painful experience. A person in whom the nerves of fingers and hands are numb may pick up a hot coffee-pot without feeling pain. This does not, however, prevent his flesh being burned to a crisp. If the pain system is effective, it corrects the problem at the cost of only a short period of suffering. On the other hand, if the system fails intellectually and emotionally to work properly, the painful experience has a tendency to spread and the "chronic-pain syndrome" is born.

As pain-feelings expand, outside influences begin to play a role. These environmental stimuli do not actually threaten harm to the body but are merely imagined to do so. People and events in our social environment may become the source of further sensory stimulation that we perceive as painful, and such influences tend to perpetuate our suffering. We can say then that chronic pain (as opposed to acute pain) is not a consequence of continuous painful impulses being received from the periphery of the body along our nerve pathways. Rather, it is a failure of the intelligent power of the brain to control and properly interpret various sensory data.

Man is in an ever-changing relationship with both his inner and outer environments. His inner environment may be thought of as having at least four closely related compartments: biological processes, sensory perceptions and motor activities, emotional drives, and intellectual functions. The four inner compartments in turn continuously relate to pressures and vacuums in the outer environment, with its great number of natural, social, and cultural variables. We are "at ease" when we are in a balanced equilibrium with both environments; we feel "diseased" when such an equilibrium, as we have learned to perceive it, is upset. The experience of pain is directly linked to such an upset.

Clearly, man has the peculiar ability to distort the marvelous survival tool nature has given him. History and daily observation tell us that man has used his intelligence not to survive but rather to destroy himself in endless, useless suffering. On the material level, man is the only creature that overeats, overdrinks, and overdrugs himself to death. Each of the various destructive habits man has learned acts as a stumbling block to his intelligent solution of problems. Such habits program the mind-body failure that often is seen as chronic pain: They deprive the chronic sufferer of coping skills needed by all of us in daily life.

To illustrate how chronic pain can occur when an injury is compounded by emotional and other influences, let's consider the case of Charlie K.

As a young man, Charlie hurts his foot playing tennis, goes to his doctor, and the x-ray studies show he has broken his ankle. The injury produces some well-defined biological changes plus a deep, throbbing discomfort in his foot. Charlie has to cut back his activities and stop playing tennis for a few weeks until the fracture has healed.

The disruption of Charlie's favorite sport along with his discomfort and the limitations on his schedule at home and work upset him emotionally and make him grouchy. His emotional suffering causes the original deep throb in his broken ankle to increase; his entire daily routine is altered by this minor fracture. Happily, he is able to adjust to the changes in his life without lasting damage to his personality and self-awareness. The fracture heals quickly, and Charlie soon returns to his previous state of healthy equilibrium. He has suffered, but has overcome, an episode of acute pain.

Fifteen years later Charlie hurts his foot again and suffers another broken ankle. By this time several changes have taken place in his life. He has gained twenty pounds. He is having a hard time maintaining his old performance levels in his favorite sport; he has been losing ground as the recognized champion of the tennis club. He is also finding it difficult to cope with the pressures of his job, and he suspects he has reached the highest plateau of his career and will not receive any more promotions.

Even before he hurt his foot, there were tensions in his

environment: He is not really "at ease" within himself. His broken ankle triggers the expected deep throbbing discomfort, but this time its meaning is completely different from that of the previous injury. The new experience is more terrifying, or anxiety-producing, since Charlie rightly suspects he will never again play tennis as he formerly did. His self-image as a youthful sportsman suffers. He becomes despondent, grouchy, withdrawn, and he fights with members of his family.

But soon he also feels a strange relief of tension: He now has a good excuse for abdicating his role as the tennis club champion—his foot "hurts too much." He finds that his constant pain keeps him from being fully proficient in his work, therefore he can be excused from duties and responsibilities he had found hard to cope with before the accident.

Now in his early fifties, Charlie K. is more unhappy than ever. He has quit his favorite sport and gained still more weight. He has managed to keep his job with adequate income, but with no prospect of further advance. He has been taking various aspirin/phenacetin compounds to control the "constant, jabbing pain" in his foot and leg, but so far he has abused no drug. However, his maladjusted personality keeps him in a chronic anxiety state, often producing feelings of anxiety and related periods of rapid breathing.

In connection with one such spell, Charlie is the victim of a car accident and suffers back pain. He is thoroughly examined in a nearby hospital and found to have "low-back sprain" for which he is put in traction for ten days and given Valium, a tranquilizing drug, in mild doses. After he is released from the hospital, he continues to complain of low-back pain and continues to take Valium. He then retains an attorney and sues the person responsible for the accident. He is examined by various specialists, and finally one surgeon decides to perform a laminectomy—a spinal operation—thinking Charlie may have a ruptured spinal disc, although no definite evidence of such a problem has been found.

Because of the surgery, Mr. K. receives various narcotic analgesic drugs and likes them. For the first time in years, he feels completely "at ease" while at the peak of narcotic action. But to continue the good feeling as tolerance develops, he needs more and more narcotic drugs. Long after he has completely recovered from the back operation, he will complain of hurt, because now he needs narcotic drugs compulsively and has learned that the best way to get his prescription refilled is to "verbalize pain." He is not malingering but is on the way to narcotic habituation and addiction.

Charlie's condition now rapidly deteriorates. He has quit work, spends all his time at home, and basically does nothing but complain. His attorney counsels him not to accept a reasonable settlement. He believes, in agreement with his lawyer, that his life has been wrecked and that he deserves a larger settlement. Pain, emotional distress, dysfunction, the desire for greater benefits from his legal claims—all these factors enormously increase his subjective feeling of suffering and misery.

He repeatedly asks his doctor for drugs and is given prescriptions for Valium and an aspirin/phenacetin compound containing codeine, to be taken four times a day when needed. Needing sedation and analgesics much more frequently, he takes the prescribed drugs every few hours, month after month. Soon he starts feeling a "burning" in his stomach, has trouble emptying his bladder, and has constipation. He is also feeling more helpless and confused, and is not able to concentrate or function well even while doing simple household chores. He is terrified and convinced he has some terrible disease, although many doctors have failed to find an organic cause for his progressively worsening condition. The more his doctors tell him that "nothing is wrong," the more frustrated he becomes, converting his frustration into physical symptoms and procuring more drug prescriptions.

Finally, one day Charlie K. is brought into the emergency room of a hospital for internal bleeding, anemia, and chronic renal failure, all of which are related to drug abuse. Weeks later he emerges from the hospital detoxified but disabled for life by chronic renal disease. He now settles his legal claim and obtains a higher monetary reward. Impaired in his ability to work, he is granted a medical retirement on Social Security disability benefits. He is fifty-two, disabled by medical "care," a man made incapable of productive work, retired ten or twelve years before retirement age because of drug misuse and a failure by society to recognize the symptoms of "conditioned pain" early enough to rehabilitate him.

The case of Charlie K. is a fictional composite of several true cases, but it is depressingly accurate. There are thousands of similar cases in the files of pain-control centers around the country: men and women, mostly middle-aged, crippled by undetected drug misuse in connection with a mismanaged chronic-pain state; human beings needlessly retired before their time for medical reasons—people who could otherwise have enjoyed productive lives for many more years.

3

How We Learn Chronic Pain and Sickness

I. P. UNIKEL

TRUE CHRONIC PAIN should not be confused with symptom-faking and malingering. People with chronic pain suffer as much as they claim they do. Their lives are as miserable as they describe them. When a painful experience is prolonged by emotional or other factors, the result can be actual biological, sensory, and motor changes, each producing further discomfort and distortion of the way one perceives things.

Our nervous system is a highly sophisticated machine. With millions of electronic-type circuits and relays, it is often compared with a computer, which continuously records input and provides related output. Like every computer, the nervous system can therefore be "programmed." If we constantly "think pain" and "talk sick," we are likely to lay the ground-work for actually being sick and miserable. There is a "learned language of pain" which involves high dramatization of pain complaints, imagery of description, and generalization of symptoms with little relation to known anatomical patterns and system organization.

We start to learn about pain and sickness at an early age. When Johnny, a first-grader, has a stomachache and is kept home from school by his parents, he is beginning to learn that certain things are not done when a person is in pain. As Johnny grows older, similar incidents occur, each strengthening the learning process.

Sooner or later, Johnny will have a reason for avoiding school. Perhaps a bully has threatened to beat him up, or he may not have studied enough for one of his exams. He tells his parents he is ill and gets to stay at home that day.

Johnny has a strong need to avoid going to school. The thought of school makes him anxious. Certainly the prospect of being physically abused by the largest boy in his class can produce such feelings. Anxiety triggers physiological responses, such as a nervous stomach, diarrhea, chest pain, dizziness, muscle cramps, and other physical symptoms.

In any case, Johnny will look for an illness that will guarantee avoidance of his problems. If he attends closely to his bodily functions, there are usually a few signs of possible sickness that he can find and embellish.

Any instance of illness, at any time in our lives, may be an occasion for learning the consequences of pain- and sickness-behavior. For example, Mrs. J. in her later years learns that she gets more attention from her husband when she is ill. She will use this to get Mr. J. to spend more time with her, stay home more, or postpone a business trip because of his concern for her. Getting attention is one of the most common consequences of learned pain-behavior. It makes such behavior more likely.

Our previous experiences, our understanding of the consequences of pain, and our particular culture are all factors in how we react to a physical disorder.

A fundamental law underlies the major principles of learning and performance. This is the "law of effect," which, simply stated, says that people tend to do things that pay off or are pleasant. If a person does something that brings a reward—that is, is followed by favorable consequences—he is more likely to behave the same way when faced again by similar circumstances. If the person's action fails to pay off or results in punishment or undesirable consequences, that behavior is less likely to recur.

For instance, a mother shows her toddler a cookie; the child says the word "cookie" and is given the treat. He will be more likely to say the word when he sees a cookie again. Being given the cookie is his reward for saying the word. On the other hand, a child who burns his hand by touching a hot stove is less likely to touch the stove a second time.

This process of association between behavior and its consequences is *learning*. Learning takes place all through our lives.

We learn about pain and sickness from our own experiences, but we also learn from the experiences of others. Pain behavior can be learned vicariously (from observing others directly), from books, television, and movies, or from being told things by others.

As noted previously, there are medical students who think they have the sicknesses they read about in their textbooks. This fact illustrates the process of suggestion that takes place when we focus carefully on our bodily processes. The medical student reads about a symptom of a dread illness in his book and tunes in on himself. If he discovers something vaguely similar, he magnifies his illness with anxiety.

There is a short comic play that dramatizes a similar example of the way pain behavior is learned. It portrays a patient who enters a reception room and waits to see the doctor because of a headache. A second patient limps into the room, and when the first patient gets up and walks over to ask the nurse a question, he also limps, although he did not do so before. This patient is clearly prone to suggestion and ends up behaving as though he were suffering the various symptoms of a half-dozen other patients who follow him into the doctor's waiting room. By now he is a mass of aches, pains, and newly acquired disabilities.

This play illustrates the power of suggestion and the fact that we learn from others how to act and to display the pain of different kinds of physical disorders. In fact, the way we talk and act is just about the only way that other people can tell we are in pain.

Three types of consequences are usually seen when people display symptoms of pain and sickness: (1) attention, (2) avoidance of stressful situations, and (3) economic advantage.

> *Attention.* It is the custom in our society to give extra attention to people who show signs of suffering. Actually, disabled people often receive more attention than they really need. They are not allowed to do things they are quite capable of doing. This is convenient for someone who has been deprived of attention during his life. This person may lack the necessary social skills to get attention or he may have a particular need for someone to lean on. Such individuals learn that they receive a lot of attention

when they are ill and when they display learned pain-behavior. They may continue to exhibit such behavior long beyond their original reason for doing so, far in excess of the actual physical causes.

Avoidance. It is relatively easy to avoid stressful situations if one has pain or is sick. Arthur L. gets chest pains every time he is supposed to speak before a group. Ruth B., a woman who was formerly admired by the men in her office, is now aging and is not receiving much attention. Rather than face her new role in the office and her advancing age, Miss B. emphasizes her pain and seeks to end her working career by claiming disability far beyond any organic causes that can be found.

Another subtle way to avoid stress is to use pain as a justification for defeat. Experts in sports medicine have pointed out that they rarely have many patients in their clinics after a winning football game. After a defeat, however, the clinic is jam-packed right after the game.

We see this same mechanism at work in people in general. Consider Robert T., a business executive who rarely demonstrates much pain behavior when he feels that he is successful and functioning well. As soon as he starts to slow down or when he experiences financial setbacks, he begins to verbalize or otherwise indicate intense pain. Mr. T. is saying, in effect, that he did not get that desired promotion or salary increase because of his backache and not because of inefficiency.

One of the typical gains of chronic-pain behavior is reduction of anxiety. Anxiety is a state of distress and physiological arousal that occurs as a response to the environment. A person engages in behaviors that reduce the anxiety or prevent its taking place. Years ago, women fainted when they were confronted by uncomfortable social situations. This, of course, had immediate anxiety-relieving consequences.

Economic Advantage. The most costly expression of learned pain-behavior in our society is that which results in economic advantage. Most obvious are the cases of malingering and outright extortion, such as those that have recently plagued the federal Workmen's Compensation program.

Case after case can be cited. Frank P. developed an exaggerated limp only when he approached a claims office. Tony R., a healthy longshoreman, collected on four successful false claims in four years. Although learning principles apply in cases such as these, the majority of patients who complain of chronic pain and sickness are far more well-meaning and the causes of their behavior are considerably more subtle and complex.

Pain behavior often leads to frequent time off from work. This process may be similar to that of Johnny staying home from school to avoid an unpleasant situation, as previously discussed. In the adult world, we see the more serious problems that result when pensions or compensations for physical disability depend on the amount of pain- or sickness-behavior the patient exhibits.

Recently, we conducted a study of patients at the Emory Pain Control Center who were receiving financial compensation for work-related injuries. We compared these patients with a similar group of patients who were receiving no compensation for chronic illness but displayed the same degree of organic disease. The patients who received compensation were significantly less likely to show improvement in a rehabilitation program. They were less likely to follow programmed instructions and had a higher dropout rate before the program was completed. Financial remuneration seems to function as a reward for learned sick-behaviors, thus insuring their continuation.

Financial incentives may also affect the patient's motivation to recover from an illness. If the financial reward for illness is greater than that for health, the person may recover much less quickly. For example, a man who earns $600 a month before taxes when he is well, and whose pension for physical disability is $450 tax-free, may not have much incentive for regaining his health. Also, a person may find considerable incentive in a financial disability payment that is less than the salary he might have earned but which involves a great deal less effort.

Because pain behavior is the way people with chronic pain and sickness have learned to meet their needs, they are highly committed to their physical complaints and resist giving them up. Their pain and sickness constitute their *raison d'être;* this is the foundation on which their behavior patterns rest.

If they give up their chronic pain and illness, they will have to learn a new behavior. To some extent, we all resist changes in our lifestyles, but chronic sufferers are especially prone to maintain their status quo. Many are neurotic and have an irrational anxiety that keeps them from solving their problems in the usual adaptive ways. Others are inadequate copers, and because of their lack of skills or declining capabilities from aging and illness, they just are not prepared to meet their needs in better ways.

Given these factors, such people constantly seek reassurance that they are in fact disabled. They constantly tell others about their pain and illness, adding considerable detail about their previous accidents and injuries and the numerous operations and other medical procedures they have endured. They make numerous visits to physicians.

For the chronic sufferer, these visits tend to be a search for justification and reaffirmation of their problems of pain and sickness, rather than attempts to obtain effective treatment and relief. Once they have learned how to show the signs of pain that achieve particular consequences for them, people increasingly rely on this behavior to meet their needs. They develop a pattern of solving problems in this fashion.

In learned pain- and sickness-behavior, however, there are losses and drawbacks as well as gains. Again, consider Johnny, who stays home from school because of illness. True, he avoids the stresses and discomforts of the classroom. But he also misses the play and good times that come after school hours, because an instant recovery would seriously endanger his status as a sufferer. Also, he may be given one or more doses of medicine and may have uncomfortable things done to him.

Johnny's adult counterpart—the chronic pain sufferer—must submit to painful shots to counteract pain, or multiple surgical operations, and spend many hours waiting in doctors' offices, or in bed, with associated discomforts and boredom.

4

The Pain-Prone Patient

I. P. UNIKEL AND
S. I. CHAPMAN

ANXIETY THAT LEADS to bodily changes and accompanying pain and physical discomfort has great significance in shaping chronic patterns of sick behavior. Physical symptoms triggered by anxiety are particularly troublesome because they themselves lead to more anxiety and its physical consequences.

Albert H. suffers anxiety when he is around women his own age. He may cross the street to avoid meeting a woman who is coming his way or behave in other strange ways. He perspires, trembles, has an increased heart rate, difficulty in breathing, dizziness, muscle tension, and loss of appetite. Sometimes he develops a headache or back and chest pains.

When Albert H. has chest pains because of anxiety, the

pains produce an even greater anxiety with more intense symptoms, such as breathing difficulties, palpitations in the chest, and a feeling of gas pressure around the heart. It is easy to see how, at this point, Albert might convince himself and others that he is having a heart attack.

Many neurotic conditions have their roots in anxiety and are relevant to a discussion of pain and illness. A common disorder is hypochondriasis, an exaggerated concern for bodily function and physical health, most frequently because of anxiety. A middle-aged person feels uncomfortable physical sensations, such as aching joints and stiffened muscles, as well as changes in appetite and sleeping habits—all resulting from aging. This leads to greater anxiety about health. If he is a hypochondriac, he worries about it, visits doctors, and may even become convinced he has a deadly disease. This often happens when he neurotically compares his own symptoms with those of friends or relatives known to have heart trouble or cancer.

But clearly, chronic-pain behavior develops because of factors other than mere anxiety about physical illness. The concepts of self-esteem and depression are useful in describing the circumstances that lead people to rely on learned pain-behavior. The way people feel about themselves is determined primarily by the extent to which their needs are being met and by whether their behavior is leading to payoffs or pleasant consequences for them. The more they achieve their desired goals, the greater their self-esteem.

Generally, depressive reactions take place when a person's needs are no longer being met. Such reactions are likely after failure and losses, such as the loss of a loved one or a good job. They are accompanied by feelings of helplessness, worthlessness, and anger at oneself. Depressed persons seldom find events around them to be pleasant.

Five categories of behavior that characterize the depressed person are: (1) statements of low self-esteem and pessimism, (2) slowed movement and poor social relationships, (3) physical complaints and self-preoccupation, (4) mental dullness and unresponsiveness, and (5) brooding and irritability.

Such behavior soon leads to troubles and maladjustment with other people and further worsens depression. Even people who are at first sympathetic with the depressed person soon learn to avoid him as much as possible. Also, depressed people often lack good social skills that win acceptance among their peers.

Almost every day we encounter situations that may lead to feelings of anxiety, helplessness, and depression. The student who works for hours and can't seem to understand anything he reads in the required advanced-calculus textbook, the person who keeps taking his car to the shop but finds it continues to run poorly, and the athlete who can't seem to make the team no matter how hard he tries—all are well acquainted with helpless feelings. These are very unpleasant. When a person first encounters a problem he can't control, he usually feels anxious and frustrated. His heart beats faster, he perspires more, his stomach becomes queasy, and he breathes more rapidly and shallowly.

This initial anxiety and frustration will often cause him to try even harder for a while. The athlete will train for long hours in hopes of making the first team; the student will hire a tutor or spend extra time studying his calculus textbook. If the extra effort is successful, the feeling of anxiety or helplessness goes away. But if it's not successful, new attitudes and behaviors are likely to develop. The person feels he is not able to control the situation and gives up: The student may make only a half-hearted effort or drop his course, the motorist may decide to buy a new car or take the bus, and the athlete may stop training and quit the team. All these solutions allow him to stop feeling anxious even though they leave him with a sense of failure.

But what if the problem has no solution and the situation is inescapable? Suppose the student has to pass calculus to stay in school, feels his whole life depends on graduating, and still can't find a way to learn the material. What happens then? Scientists have found that serious disturbances occur in people in these situations. They become very passive and depressed. In many cases, they not only stop trying to do the things they think they can't do, but they also stop doing the things they *can* do. The student quits studying English, which he had always mastered easily, or stops seeing friends and spends more time lying in bed and doing nothing. Eventually he loses perspective about what he can do. His confidence and self-esteem drop to the point that he believes he can't control any situation. Our failing student might even come to feel that he could not do well in English even if he tried; or worse, he might lose faith in his ability to do *anything* successfully.

If this feeling of total helplessness continues, it will have drastic consequences. The individual feels constantly unhappy and dissatisfied, develops feelings of uselessness and self-dislike, and believes the future is black. Nothing is enjoyable—not eating, not sex, not human companionship.

An anxious person seeks above all to engage in behavior that will reduce his anxiety. People who are failing to get important needs met and who suffer from depression and a loss of self-esteem will seek to explain failure in ways that make them look better. Pain and sickness provide a socially acceptable excuse for doubts about oneself and one's ability to cope with life and for the low self-esteem and depression that result from failure to cope successfully.

The background of pain-prone patients often includes previous learning of the sick role. The patient may have current problems, such as a bona fide physical illness, or hypochondriac tendencies. These patients, once they begin treatment, continue seeking opportunities to gain access to doctors' offices, where they continue to learn by observing physicians and other medical personnel. They also find out what other patients are doing and what behaviors are successful for them. Their learned pain-behavior thus grows.

Especially when interacting with doctors, these patients learn to say and do things that reconfirm their pain and sickness and maintain their status as sufferers and invalids. Many observers have characterized the nature of these interactions as "pain games."

A typical game is the one played by Mrs. B., a chronic patient who flatters her current doctor and is critical of previous physicians she has seen. If the doctor is not astute about learned pain-behavior, he may find that he has been manipulated into a series of unnecessary and expensive medical tests and treatments on Mrs. B. If he does so, she will praise his decision, because these procedures will continue to justify her learned pain-behavior.

There are many such games, and they all serve to perpetuate cycles of medical-treatment failure and repeated, ineffective surgery. In addition to trying to influence a particular doctor, such patients also shop around, looking for doctors who will give them what they want. In this way they are rewarded for learned pain-behavior—in other words, their pain behavior is reinforced.

An experiment done with pigeons best illustrates the process of learned helplessness, or, as it has also been called, "learned laziness." A group of pigeons was kept in a cage and given food regardless of their behavior: they were not required to perform any work or activity at all. When these experimental subjects were later placed in a situation where a response was necessary for them to obtain food, they appeared to have learned that they would be fed regardless of their behavior. They were much less capable of doing the work required for them to eat than were pigeons without similar previous experience.

It is highly possible that learned helplessness, just as in the pigeons, makes the recipient of workmen's compensation and other such payments less able to return to work after physical improvement has taken place. In other words, paying people to be sick seems to make it harder and less likely for them to be rehabilitated, no matter how honest their intentions.

Pain-prone patients (or chronic sufferers) most frequently are neurotic, with anxiety and tension. Under stress, they are likely to break down with psychosomatic illnesses. They have physical symptoms, such as back and chest pain and headaches, which serve to reduce anxiety and help them meet their immediate needs by securing attention or getting them out of stressful situations. They have "learned" pain behavior. Their symptoms in a large number of cases will eventually bring them economic advantages.

Such patients tend to be passive and dependent on

others for emotional and financial support. They are usually depressed, in which case they show disgust, discouragement, irritability, tiredness, slowing down, feeling sorry for themselves, and despair.

Their anxiety is high but they tend to deny or fail to recognize their emotional problems. They find physical, organic explanations more acceptable and compatible with their self-concepts than emotional reasons.

Behaviorally, they verbalize an extensive and varied number of physical complaints and consume large quantities of pills throughout the day, as the urge to do so strikes them.

They spend a significant amount of time in doctors' offices and medical facilities. They limit their activities and stay in bed much of the time, because of the presumed dangers of trying to get up and lead a normal life. They are thus able to avoid social encounters and sexual relations, even those that previously brought them pleasure. In general, their lives are far from pleasant: They are truly sufferers.

5

Pain and Drug Misuse

S. F. BRENA

NO MODERN SOLDIER could stand the suffering of Americans who fought in the War between the States, when limbs were amputated under a mere buffer of chloroform, and little morphine was available to reduce pain after surgery. No antibiotic was then available to reduce the agony of infection, gangrene, intestinal diseases, and the pneumonia that killed the hero of the South, Stonewall Jackson, after his arm was amputated.

Have we genetically and neurologically changed from our forefathers? Not likely. Rather, we have been conditioned by psychological manipulation and social learning to reject the experience of pain from our lives.

One example of this is the way the pharmaceutical industry has talked us into believing drugs can solve all our problems, relieve our aches and pains, and give us nightly the bliss of sleep. We believe this no matter how badly we mistreat our bodies and overburden our minds with worry. What the industry does not tell us, and what physicians themselves often fail to remember, is the dreadful price we pay in terms of drug intoxication.

Chronic drug-intake leads to emotional habituation and dependence on drugs as a way of life. Every day, thousands of tons of aspirin, tranquilizers, sleeping pills, and antihistamines are gulped down in this country. Americans also spend an estimated $10 billion a year on alcohol and smoke six hundred billion cigarettes a year, forgetting that alcohol and nicotine are poisonous drugs.

Today's society has abandoned many of the older rules and customs concerning drugs, and this departure has had a profound and dangerous impact on Western culture. In nineteenth-century America, genteel ladies could discreetly use a mild combination of alcohol and opium, called laudanum, to calm their menstrual discomfort, but they were frowned on if caught taking the drug too often and too openly. It was also considered unmanly for an early-American gentleman to show drug dependence in connection with chronic-pain complaints.

We label as medical problems today a large number of conditions once viewed as the normal trials of human existence. We take it for granted that drugs should be prescribed and widely used to deal with interpersonal situations and emotional pressures. Since a medical label is tagged to these strains and tensions, the shame of social disapproval no longer hinders drug abusers. In some ways, we've become "allergic" to pain. Once learning is accomplished and the label "pain" is presented to our neurotic behavior, this simple, abstract English word is likely to arouse more emotions, more concern, and more attention than any other in our vocabulary.

The use of drugs to lessen pain is one of the oldest forms of medical practice. In the Code of Hammurabi, a document of the great civilization that flourished in Mesopotamia between 3,000 and 2,000 B.C., eleven out of 282 paragraphs refer to the practices of physicians and veterinarians. Many drugs are mentioned in these ancient writings, among them hyosciamus, hellebore, mandrake, opium, and belladonna.

All of these drugs are known to have some pain-relieving effects. The same drugs are mentioned again in both the Edwin Smith and Ebers papyri which describe the medical practices of ancient Egypt. Opium, in fact, is described as a remedy of divine origin prescribed by Isis for curing the Pharaoh's headaches. The writings of later famous physicians such as Diosconides, Pliny the Elder, Galen, and Avicenna contain numerous prescriptions of herbs and drugs for the relief of various aches and ailments.

One of the common ways the ancients lessened pain from severe injury was to induce sleep by having the patient inhale the fumes of burning hemp. Another way was to soak a common sea sponge in a mixture of opium, hyoscine, and mandragora juices: the so-called somniferous sponge of the Middle Ages. Remedies used in ancient and medieval times were unpredictable, empirical, and often harmful. More than once they must have helped to relieve pain permanently by inducing the final sleep of death.

Man's history is full of examples in which the fear of death must have overshadowed the agony of pain. Patients underwent painful surgeries such as the amputation of extremities without first being rendered unconscious. One of the last of these dreadful surgeries, which occurred shortly before the advent of modern anesthesia with ether and chloroform, is described by the Italian writer Silvio Pellico. In his book, *Le Mie Prigioni,* published in the first part of the nineteenth century, he vividly describes the amputation of a gangrenous leg. The patient is Pietro Maroncelli, a political prisoner held in the infamous Spielberg prison in Austria.

While the Austrian surgeon is still working on the bloody stump of the amputated limb, Maroncelli, fully awake, is quoted as saying to the surgeon: "Thank you, sir. You have just liberated me from a dangerous enemy. Being a prisoner, I have little but a flower to offer you in appreciation." What an impressive example of self-control and positive thinking!

Before the onset of present-day knowledge of drugs, remedies for pain were prescribed in minimal doses, well below what now is considered safe. Drugs were prescribed more for a magical than a chemical action. Today we call the "magical" action of drugs a "placebo" effect, which means that the drug works by virtue of the patient's own expectation and desire to be relieved, rather than by its own chemical effectiveness.

Every health professional discovers the crucial importance of the placebo effect in drug action and interaction. The art of using it can allow minimum doses to be given with enhanced beneficial effects on patients. The American Medical Association has long recognized the placebo effect. Many research studies have been designed to better understand the proper role of this powerful therapeutic tool.

But the fact remains, "Poison is in every drug, and nothing is without poison; the dosage makes it either a poison or a remedy." This was written by the physician Paracelsus centuries ago. In acute life- or health-threatening situations, whether from injury or disease, it is correct and safe to use drugs in proper doses to take care of the emergency and to reduce the related anxiety and pain.

However, the situation changes when the same drugs are used to control chronic pain. For example, long-term administration of drugs can stimulate the activity of certain liver enzymes, with unexpected consequences. The duration of a drug's action—the barbiturate in a sleeping pill, for instance—is diminished by prolonged usage, so that rapidly increasing doses are needed to achieve sleep. This phenomenon is called tachyphylaxis. Eventually, the point is reached where not much sleep is induced even by enormous amounts of the barbiturate, and meanwhile, the poisonous effects of the drug have skyrocketed.

In a patient who regularly abuses one drug, the duration of action of an unrelated drug may also be reduced, since the liver enzymes affected are not specific. The patient may fail to respond to this second drug in a time of emergency, when it may be a matter of saving his life. Patients abusing barbiturates, for example, can also develop tolerance to dicumarol, a chemical that reduces blood coagulation. Such patients may fail to respond to dicumarol when confronted by a deadly pulmonary embolus.

Four groups of chemicals are known to have some usefulness in pain management: (1) salicylates, (2) opiates, (3) barbiturates, and (4) tranquilizers. Let's look at some of the hazards of chronic misuse of these drugs.

Salicylates. The bark of the willow tree (*Salix alba*) contains a salicyl alcohol that for centuries has been known to decrease fevers. Not until 1875, however, was a synthetic salicylate salt made available with properties similar to those of the bark of a willow tree. In 1899 another chemical compound, the acetyl ester of salicyl acid, was introduced as the first preparation of the drug in the solid form of tablets: This new product was called aspirin.

Aspirin not only effectively relieves pain, it also reduces fever and helps many inflammatory processes. It does this probably by reducing the swelling of joints and other inflamed body tissues. The most successful use of aspirin is in the treatment of various rheumatic and arthritic disorders as well as in the control of headaches caused by tension.

If taken within prescribed limits and not constantly in high doses, aspirin is a relatively safe drug. However, when a patient abuses aspirin, harm can result. The best known of these effects is stomach upset; the aggravation of gastritis and ulcer symptoms by aspirin can lead to stomach bleeding and the undetected loss of blood in stools. Aspirin in large doses can also affect the liver, resulting in defects of blood-clotting mechanisms and metabolic functions, with loss of such important substances as amino acids through the kidneys. The respiratory system may be affected, resulting in increased rates of breathing.

By far the most frightening symptoms of aspirin toxicity are those affecting the nervous system: dizziness, ringing in the ears, drowsiness, visual disturbances, and deafness. Often the patient doesn't connect these symptoms with chronic aspirin-abuse and becomes anxious and upset, fearing he may have a serious brain lesion, perhaps even brain cancer.

Expensive medical studies are sometimes done needlessly because a patient fails to tell his doctor he is taking large doses of aspirin. The physician himself may neglect to ask the proper questions and may not recognize the more subtle symptoms of aspirin toxicity.

One reason for these misunderstandings is the way the

mass media publicize drugs sold over the counter without medical prescription, claiming they will relieve aches and pains of every kind. The chronic sufferer always searches for a "magic" drug to stop his pains. He is an easy target for media campaigns proclaiming that a certain drug has "more pain-relieving effects" than its competitors.

What the uninformed customer does not know is that many popular remedies sold as pain relievers contain a combination of aspirin and phenacetin plus various other ingredients with no proven analgesic action. In therapeutic doses, phenacetin is an effective pain-relieving drug matching the action of aspirin. However, phenacetin in large doses is known to produce anemia, skin rashes, and kidney damage.

Because he lacks proper information, the chronic sufferer may buy various popular drugs with different brand-names. He thinks he is taking different remedies, when actually they are the same mixtures. Unknown to himself and undetected by his physician, toxicity from aspirin and phenacetin may build up and lead to chronic kidney disease and kidney failure. In turn, kidney disease usually produces pain and discomfort in the flank and back regions. The pain is disturbing and likely to increase the patient's demand for drugs; thus we see one of the most subtle and harmful "vicious cycles" of pain and disease.

Years ago, when I was working with the pain team at the University Hospital in Seattle, a patient was referred to the pain clinic for treatment of "intractable" cancer pain. She had had a cancer of the bowel removed a year earlier, and no sign of cancer diffusion was ever found in repeated and careful medical follow-ups. The patient, however, was convinced she was dying in agony because of cancer and stayed in bed around the clock.

She arrived at the hospital in an ambulance, and the first thing she told the doctor was: "I'm going to die very soon! I already hear the bells of heaven ringing in my ears!" Of course she did; she was taking 15–20 tablets of aspirin No. 4 each day, containing one grain of codeine per tablet, which made her dizzy and unable to stand. After she was detoxified, she got out of bed, took physical-therapy exercises and psychological counseling, and finally became convinced she did not have diffused cancer. This sufferer, who had come to the hospital in an ambulance, left three weeks later on her feet and went immediately to enjoy a good meal at one of Seattle's best restaurants.

In the last few years, the pharmaceutical industry has become aware of the dangers of aspirin misuse, and has successfully marketed a number of drugs claiming they can provide pain relief without the dangers of aspirin. The chemical most commonly used in such "aspirin-free" preparations is acetaminophen which is similar to phenacetin, with less renal toxicity. The best known and most widely prescribed aspirin-free pain-killer drug is Tylenol, a good and mild nonopiate analgesic drug. However, the pharmaceutical industry fails to clearly inform its customers that compounds containing acetaminophen, such as Tylenol, do not have the anti-inflammatory action of the salicylates, which is so often useful to relieve the discomfort associated with the inflamed joints of the patient with acute arthritis; nor does it warn of the danger of acetaminophen abuse which can severely damage certain cells of the liver.

Opiates. Many compounds are included in this group of drugs, all with similar characteristic features. They include natural derivatives of opium, such as morphine and codeine; chemical derivatives of morphine and codeine, such as heroin; synthetic opiates, such as pethidine (Demerol) and methadone.

The poet Homer probably described the first historically recorded use of opiates in the *Iliad,* when he wrote that "Helen cast a drug into the wine . . . to lull all pain and anger, and bring every sorrow into oblivion." This Homeric verse describes the various useful effects of opiate intake: relief of pain, relaxation of anxiety, sedation, drowsiness, and sleep.

Actually, scientists were in the dark until recently about the properties of opiates. Do opiates act on the whole brain, depressing it into chemical submission? Or do they act on specialized brain regions, on sites called opiate-receptors in the brain's nerve cells?

Strong evidence now favors the opiate-receptor theory. The existence of specialized nerve cells with a high sensitivity to opiates makes it easy to better understand the mode of action of morphine, but on the other hand, the presence of these specialized nerve cells raises an entirely new set of questions.

Why should the brain have cells sensitive to chemical compounds like opiates, which are not manufactured by the body? A common-sense hypothesis is that the brain's opiate-receptors developed because of some opiate-like substance made inside the body itself. Morphine just happens to be similar to this substance in its effects on the nervous system. Once the hypothesis was made, a race began to find this substance inside the body; it was won in 1975 by a research team in Scotland. John Hughes and Hans W. Kosterlitz at the University of Aberdeen reported finding a chemical in a specially prepared extract of pig's brain that seemed to produce effects similar to those of morphine when placed on the pig's opiate-receptors.

They called the newly discovered brain substance enkephalin.

The potential consequences of the discovery of enkephalin are far-reaching, but as of this writing the new chemical has not been developed for clinical applications in medicine. An interesting sidelight is that brain morphine-receptors have been found densely clustered around certain specific brain areas, such as the limbic region—the so-called visceral brain, known to be associated with the physical expression of emotional forces. This information suggests that one important action of morphine in controlling pain may be to relieve emotional pressures by helping block conversion of emotional factors into bodily discomfort.

Opiates are useful drugs when used for short periods to control acute pain from actual injury or disease. However, they are a serious cause of complications and unending misery when used over long periods in chronic-pain situations. Tolerance to opiates grows rapidly. In a few days, larger doses may be required to produce the same pain-relieving effects.

When patients are at peak opiate action, they "feel great." When their opiate blood levels are low, they feel miserable and take another tablet or shot. They justify their drug needs with complaints of high-intensity pain. As tolerance builds, the interval between each subsequent peak action is progressively shortened to the point where patients must take the drug almost constantly to avoid unpleasant withdrawal symptoms.

Another effect is that tolerance to one opiate produces a cross-tolerance to all other opiates. This is unfortunate and most damaging when a terminal cancer patient is involved. If opiate intake unwisely has been started too early in the progress of cancer, the patient may have cross-tolerance to all opiates by the time the disease has evolved into its terminal and painful stage of metastatic diffusion.

Cross-tolerance can be overcome only by withdrawing the patient from all opiates for a while or by constantly increasing the dosage. The second alternative, however, is likely to compound the harmful side-effects of opiates, such as constipation, urinary retention, constriction of the lung's air passages, and low blood-pressure.

The most commonly prescribed opiate for the control of chronic pain is codeine, a short-acting drug only one-tenth as potent a pain-killer as morphine. To supplement its potency, codeine is often mixed with aspirin and phenacetin in the compounds labeled No. 2 (one-fourth grain of codeine), No. 3 (one-half grain), and No. 4 (one grain). As tolerance builds with use, patients tend to increase the doses to obtain more codeine, but in the process they also take increased doses of aspirin and phenacetin, to the point where kidney damage may develop.

In addition to kidney lesions, codeine-induced urinary retention sets a favorable stage for chronic urinary-tract infection. The result may be a crippled patient with a serious, potentially life-threatening, iatrogenic disease (*iatrogenic* in Greek means "produced by a physician"). Large numbers of chronic sufferers with long histories of drug abuse show evidence of chronic, unexplained urinary infection for which continuing medical care and prescription of antibiotics have become mandatory.

A weak, opiate-like chemical with low addiction liability is propoxyphene, best known to the American customer as Darvon. The real pain-relieving action of Darvon is no better than aspirin, and yet Darvon is widely prescribed over aspirin preparations, despite the fact that it costs more and that it shares some of the dangers of opiate addiction. Darvon is also frequently associated in compounds containing aspirin and phenacetin, with the added risks of toxicity when abused, but with no greater actual analgesic action.

Barbiturates. These drugs do not have any direct pain-relieving effect. They act mainly to depress the central nervous system, producing sedation and sleep. They are frequently prescribed to help patients with chronic pain and related anxiety-depression to fall asleep. However, this artificially induced sleep heavily taxes the general welfare of the individual.

Barbiturates produce sedation and sleep through a mechanism that is basically a poisoning of the nervous system by interfering with the proper oxygenation of the brain and nerve cells. Research has shown that brain cells decrease their activity nearly to a standstill while under the influence of a barbiturate. As soon as blood levels of the chemical are reduced by eliminating the drug from the body, the brain cells start to "fire" again, but in such a disorderly fashion as to mimic a seizure.

In fact, attacks of epileptic-like seizures are a common life-threatening feature of the barbiturate-withdrawal syndrome. When nerve cells start firing in a disorderly, seizure-like manner, a peculiar, highly unpleasant feeling of restlessness, nervousness, and muscular twitches and spasms is perceived. This compels the patient to take another barbiturate tablet, with addiction soon resulting.

The most damaging barbiturate compounds are those in which the drug is mixed with aspirin and phenacetin to relieve pain while helping the patient fall asleep. The uninformed patient may take such a compound several times a day, trying to control his habitual pain and the "muscle spasms" that constantly bother him.

The outcome is chronic impairment of reasoning and judgment, inefficiency at work, distractability, distorted reaction-time, and wrecked motor-coordination. All of this leads to a likelihood of vehicle and on-the-job accidents. In tracing the medical histories of patients disabled by a traffic or a work injury, a pattern of barbiturate abuse for sleep and chronic-pain problems is often documented.

Tranquilizing drugs. Barbiturates and bromides were used widely in the past to provide relief from emotional tension. Their use for these purposes has recently been decreased in favor of other groups of drugs that seem to act more selectively on the limbic system, providing a tranquilizing action without the generalized depressive effects that the barbiturates have on the brain.

Among the many drugs used to treat states of emotional tension and anxiety, one group has emerged as the favorite of all prescriptions for tranquilizers. These are the benzodiazepines, which include diazepam (Valium) and chlordiazepoxide (Librium). When properly used in acute and semiacute short-lived anxiety states, as in the tension felt in association with surgery or with a trauma, Valium and Librium are excellent medications capable of providing relaxation and a pleasant feeling of well-being. When taken over long periods, however, these drugs, like all remedies, cause a tolerance which requires higher doses to achieve the same pleasant effects.

A large dose of Valium produces drowsiness, uncoordinated movements, and impairment of judgment and performance similar to the effects of barbiturates. One of the risks of Valium intake is that equal doses of the drug affect different individuals in different ways. Some patients may incur dangerous mental and motor impairments on very small doses of Valium. This, if not detected, can seriously expose the Valium-user to the risk of accidents. Other dangerous effects of Valium are skin rashes and muscle tenderness, both of which cause distress to the patient and make him likely to take drugs. Generalized seizures are sometimes seen in Valium withdrawal, as they are in barbiturate withdrawal.

Valium, one of the most widely prescribed drugs in the United States, is often given for chronic-pain conditions. Yet experience has shown that, paradoxically, the drug seems to increase the subjective pain experience, possibly through a feeling of confusion and helplessness. Most of the patients abusing Valium for chronic pain agree that they feel much better when the drug dependence has been eliminated and Valium use discontinued.

After spending twenty years working with people in pain, I have found that undetected drug abuse is the single most devastating complication in chronic-pain cases. It is a problem that condemns millions of people to a lifetime of unnecessary misery, dysfunction, and disability.

6

Pain and Surgery

W. D. HAMMONDS

MUCH OF THE PAIN that doctors see in pain clinics is either produced or made worse by medical treatment. This includes surgery that is too often unnecessary or even harmful. Many of these surgical procedures are applied to the nervous system, which is intimately associated with our perception of pain.

Two nations with similar backgrounds and lifestyles, such as the United States and Great Britain, would normally be expected to have a similar incidence of surgically treatable diseases. Yet twice as much surgery is performed on a per capita basis each year in the United States as in Great Britain. There is one operation per thirteen people in this country and only one per twenty-six in England and Wales. It is not surprising, then, that, again on a per capita basis, there are twice as many surgeons in the United States as in Great Britain. This suggests the grim "law" that the number of operations expands to meet the case-load needs of available surgeons.

There are also statistics to show that the number of both operations and surgeons rises with the wealth of an area's residents and the number of hospital beds available. This tells us that the decision to operate or not to operate is influenced by economic factors rather than by specific criteria for surgery based on the patient's disease. In fact, one highly publicized study has shown that when a second opinion from another surgeon was obtained, about 24 percent of elective operations were deemed unnecessary.

Fads abound in surgery. A few years ago tonsillectomy was one of the most commonly performed procedures, but in recent years the number of tonsillectomies has decreased by one third. Downward trends such as these cast doubt on the need for certain operations. To be sure, there are situations in which the best scientific knowledge, based on objective criteria, unanimously indicates the need for surgery, but in many circumstances, there is a great deal of room for doubt.

For example, some women develop an overwhelming fear of having more children. It is obvious to them on a conscious level that a hysterectomy would relieve them of this worry forever. Unconsciously, they begin to verbalize and actually suffer the symptoms they have come to associate with disorders of the uterus from talking with their peers. They develop pelvic fullness, heavy periods, and nagging backache.

The surgeon, meanwhile, needs to keep his surgical case-load high: A busy surgeon is a successful surgeon. He wants to do what he was trained to do, and a fee-for-service method of paying for medical care makes surgical procedures very profitable.

So the conversation in the surgeon's office often goes something like this: *Doctor:* "I can't promise you that a hysterectomy would relieve your back pain." *Mrs. J.:* "I'm so desperate to get rid of this pain I'm willing to take that chance." This interchange soothes the surgeon's conscience. For his own decision-making process, the fact that upon examination the patient has a completely normal uterus becomes less important.

Mrs. J. has suppressed the fact that her unconscious desire for permanent birth control is the origin of her symptoms. This is not to condemn surgical birth control, but there are safer methods. Surgery has risks of bleeding, infection, and damage to other organs. Anesthesia, necessary for the surgery, carries with it risks of heart, lung, and other complications that are potentially lethal.

The Mrs. J. incident helps explain why so much surgery that is unnecessary on the basis of strictest scientific data is being performed today. The patient virtually "asks for it," and the surgeon is either consciously or unconsciously influenced by the fee. Also, as in the example just cited, pain plays a large part in the decision to perform surgery. Pain is such a completely subjective symptom that it has never been measured adequately enough to allow its inclusion in the strictest scientific criteria for surgery.

One of the hottest controversies in medicine today has to do with surgery for a disease in which pain is a major symptom. The issue is whether there is need for heart surgery in patients with blockage of the blood supply to the heart. Narrowing of the heart's vessels is one of the leading causes of death in American men; several years ago an operation was developed in which the blocked segments of the heart's arteries are bypassed with veins taken from elsewhere in the patient's body. This was a novel idea, but the evidence that it prolongs life is inconclusive. One of the main reasons that heart-bypass surgery continues to be performed and is growing in popularity is that chest pain associated with heart disease often disappears after this procedure.

These results may be misleading, however. Because pain is so difficult to measure, it can confuse the rational scientific approach. Several years ago another surgical way of dealing with this kind of heart disease was devised, in which blood from other vessels was diverted to the heart. This procedure also had as one of its outstanding results the relief of pain. In a controlled study, half of the patients who presented themselves with this kind of heart disease had the surgical procedure performed, while the remainder merely had their chests opened and closed without doing any further surgical procedure. The patients were all told that the surgery had been done. The results in relieving pain were exactly the same.

In today's world of patients having to give their informed consent, the study just prescribed could not be done, but we can still wonder if pain would be relieved by a minor skin incision across the chest as effectively as by heart-bypass surgery.

In any event, in most areas of medicine, the cards are stacked in such a way that patients have a good chance of getting unnecessary surgery. The odds are weighted most heavily against the patient in chronic-pain cases.

In one of the most common kinds of chronic pain—low-back pain—surgical treatment began on an optimistic note in 1934, when W. J. Mixer and J. S. Barr reported dramatic relief of pain after removal of protruding bits of disc tissue. The disc is a cushion of padding between two vertebrae; the center of this cushion is soft, and sometimes, because of added pressure on the disc and for other reasons that are poorly understood, the soft center ruptures through the margins of the disc and comes to rest against spinal nerves. This ruptured disc causes pain as it presses against nerves leaving the spinal column.

Since back pain is such a common problem, it is not surprising that surgeons should want to use spinal surgery to obtain dramatic relief for patients who clamor for relief. As with many new surgical techniques, disc surgery was first performed on patients with overwhelming physical symptoms, but as success stories spread, the operation began to be performed on patients with "back pain" but without physically measurable indications for surgery.

The problem is that back pain is not always caused by something as straightforward as a ruptured disc. The people who do have a ruptured disc can be cured by early operation, but most patients have other causes of their back pain; this group will not be helped and may be harmed by surgery. Acute back-pain can be caused by a recently ruptured disc, while chronic pain can arise from a multitude of sources: It has strong elements of learned behavior in it.

Back pain is so common that the person with an emotional need for pain has models all around him to learn from. The patient may unconsciously pattern his learned pain-behavior after an older sibling or father-figure who suffers from back pain. When such a pattern of chronic-pain behavior is established, the stage is set for later surgery by the procedure-oriented surgeon who will do harm instead of helping the patient.

In light of this background, it is not surprising that such poor results have been recorded in the surgical treatment of low-back pain. A report published in the *Canadian Medical Association Journal* showed that the rate of success for all surgical operations of this type was between

30 percent and 40 percent. By contrast, the rate of satisfactory results in conservatively treated patients who had had no surgery was 75 percent.

The best results in back surgery seem to be obtained in an initial operation when there are definite symptoms of physical disease of recent onset, a physical defect can be located on x-rays, and the defect relates to the distribution of pain. Second operations are less successful, and third and fourth procedures are much less so. Nonetheless, we continue to see patients in the Emory Pain Control Center who have had five or six back operations. Dr. S. F. Brena has seen several patients who have had more than ten back operations, while the record may be held by a man in Seattle who endured twenty-one surgical procedures for back pain.

Dorsal rhizotomy is a neurosurgical procedure in which the surgeon cuts the roots of the nerves connecting the spinal cord with a specific part of the anatomy. Some of the nerve fibers in these roots traditionally have been associated with pain. But again, the application of this procedure to patients has not brought encouraging results. Eminently qualified neurosurgeons achieved only a 28 percent long-term success rate when this operation was performed for chronic pain.

If failure to cure is not indictment enough, it is also recognized that after a rhizotomy, patients are often afflicted with burning pains in that part of the body served by the cut nerves.

Cordotomy, a surgical division of that quadrant of the spinal cord traditionally thought to carry painful impulses, is another neurosurgical procedure used and overused to treat chronic pain. The idea goes back to 1905, when a Dr. Spiller observed that a patient dying of widespread tuberculosis had lost pain-and-temperature sensation in the lower part of his body. When the patient died, it was learned on autopsy that the tuberculosis infection had destroyed certain nerve tracts which are clustered in a particular section of the spinal cord.

In 1911, Spiller persuaded a surgeon, Dr. Martin, to divide this part of the spinal cord in a patient with severe pain of the lower extremity caused by an incurable tumor of the spine. The surgery was a partial success, and many such operations have since been performed.

But cordotomy, like rhizotomy, is associated with burning pain in the denervated area of the body. It also can be associated with loss of the ability to control the bladder and bowels. Despite these frightening side-effects, this procedure is performed too many times each year, and in chronic pain the results are very poor.

Why are operations that are anatomically correct so often followed by poor results? The reasons are clearly found in the vast differences between acute and chronic pain.

Acute pain does follow traditional anatomic pathways; it is the kind of pain that allows us to protect ourselves from injury if we touch a hot stove by accident. Acute pain can be decreased by blocking the appropriate pain-conveying fibers and pathways. Acute pain is not a disabling problem that is difficult to treat; it is a healthy signal that tells us something is wrong with our body.

But after pain is endured for three or four months, it may cease to be acute pain and become the chronic pain that is perpetuated by emotional factors, by learned patterns of behavior, by conscious or unconscious secondary gains, and as a means of justifying the continued use of drugs without having to assume personal responsibility. This is the pain against which surgical procedures are often useless.

Today's surgeons must establish criteria for the performance of surgery that take into consideration new knowledge about the behavioral and emotional aspects of chronic pain. And they would do well to accept the wisdom of their own truism: "When you operate for pain, you seldom find it."

7

Ways and Attempts to Measure Pain

S. F. BRENA

PHYSICIANS SOMETIMES exchange telephone calls such as: "Will you examine a patient of mine? He's in terrible pain, but I can't find a disease to explain it." Or: "Will you admit a patient of mine to your service? She's been suffering for three years, and now she's in real agony and I can't understand why."

What does it mean when a patient has "terrible pain?" Does he have cancer? Is he suffering from heart disease? Is he in the agony of drug addiction? Or is he having problems with his wife, his boss, his in-laws? Does he have a suit pending that will soon come up in court, the prospect of which has turned him into a neurotically sick individual?

If chronic pain could be measured accurately, the answers to these questions might be found more quickly. I and many of my colleagues believe it is possible to measure chronic pain. Yet the problems in doing so are formidable, because the pain is intimately tied to the sufferer's emotions and other nonphysical factors. Indeed, the cynical observer might compare the effort to trying to measure grief, rage, or love.

A satisfactory pain indicator would be a measurable body function which is present or increased when pain is perceived, and absent or decreased when pain is not present, just as changes in the blood levels of oxygen, carbon dioxide, and lactates are a good sign of how well we are breathing. For instance, we know the liver regulates certain enzymes that can be measured; a change in the blood levels of these enzymes can be viewed as an indication of a liver disorder.

No such physiological indicator now available will measure clinical pain exactly. But efforts are being made to design more reliable and easy-to-communicate systems of pain measurement.

The German philosopher Leibniz stated in his theory of the "monad" centuries ago that each person is a monad—a complete, closed system, separate from outer experience unless he engages in some form of communication with the outside world. We are all like "black boxes" and what goes on inside the black box, no observer can tell.

However, the observer can make statements about what goes into the black box (input) and what comes out (output). So the example of the black box can be used to design a system for the measurement of pain. Even though we can't measure the subjective feeling of pain, we can accurately measure events related to the pain experience and set a standard of rules by which numbers can be assigned to such events.

Most events which can be numbered in the measurement of pain are behavioral. As an example, when we feel pain we tend to complain and show various changes in our outward behavior: these are responses of the whole organism, and they can be recorded and numerically assessed.

If a person is subject to an intensely painful stimulus which causes a change in blood pressure, this blood pressure change can also be operationally defined as a pain response and some of its characteristics measured: The degree of variation from the pre-stimulus level can be expressed in millimeters of mercury. If we apply electrodes on the skin of a patient's back region, then stimulate him with a pin-prick sharp enough to produce a movement of the spine, a set of impulses will be seen on an electronic oscilloscope. These impulses can be recorded, measured, and averaged. They are an effective way to measure muscular responses to a painful stimulus.

Traditionally, clinical pain has been defined in terms of verbal complaints which have been viewed as accurate indicators of degrees of painful stimulation from a disease process. However, many scientists question the validity of pain complaints as measures of pathologic states. They challenge the common belief that how loudly a patient cries or how frequently his "sick talk" comes can be taken as measurements of pain perception.

Researchers over the past five decades have used the concept of the "pain threshold," defined as the lowest perceivable experience of pain caused by a stimulus that represents the least amount of stimulation necessary to elicit an observable response. Using the familiar cuff of the instrument for measuring blood pressure, for instance, it can be said that the pain threshold of a certain individual is 140 if he displays a pain response when the cuff is inflated to 140 millimeters of mercury pressure.

Pain thresholds are useful research tools but are difficult to interpret on clinical grounds. This is because of the trouble we have connecting a threshold stimulus with the individual's reaction as a whole and the amount of detectable damage in bodily organs and systems.

Richard A. Sternbach and his colleagues have designed a newer technique for measuring clinical pain, based on the threshold model. This measures the maximum length of time a subject can tolerate a discomfort produced when he squeezes a hand-exerciser continuously while a tourniquet or an overinflated blood-pressure cuff is applied to one of his arms. As time goes by, the subject becomes increasingly uncomfortable and is instructed to stop when he can no longer tolerate the discomfort. He is also asked to indicate when the level of his discomfort matches his habitual clinical-pain experience. By this arrangement, an investigator can not only measure pain threshold but also the *ratio* between a person's perceived habitual-pain intensity and his pain threshold.

For example, the pain ratio would be one-to-two if a person said his habitual pain experience was matched after five minutes of squeezing the hand-exerciser, but he could continue the procedure for ten minutes before he could no longer tolerate the tourniquet discomfort. Pain ratio is a useful reference point by which the subjective feeling of pain can be assessed.

Various "paper-and-pencil" tests have been designed to measure different types of sick behaviors. Best known is the Minnesota Multiphasic Personality Inventory (MMPI), which is a measure of psychological adjustment. Research has shown that certain psychological profiles in the MMPI test do portray the pain-prone patient as described in Chapter Four.

Other paper-and-pencil tests assign numbers to a patient's complaints about pain. The McGill Pain Questionnaire has earned good acceptance among clinicians for its accuracy. This questionnaire includes groups of words that patients often use to describe their pain experience. These words are grouped into categories, each representing a dimension of pain experience.

For example, one dimension relates to fear, and the words are "fearful, frightening, terrifying." The subject is instructed to circle on the questionnaire the word that best describes his pain. The words are rated according to intensity of the pain they represent; in the above example, "terrifying" is a more intense description than "fearful." The McGill Pain Questionnaire tells the practitioner how a patient perceives his pain. The data can be compared with objective findings of a physical examination to see how closely the patient's reported pain experience fits with objective evidence of a disease process. The questionnaire can also help evaluate the effectiveness of a pain-treatment program from the patient's point of view.

Performance tests are also useful in the measurement of chronic-pain states. One objective performance test is "joint goniometry." This measures the ranges of motion of various joints by using a goniometer, an instrument that establishes exact degrees of angulation. Routine physical activity, an important behavioral dimension of pain, can be monitored by diary-type questionnaires on which the sufferer is requested to record how much time he devotes to simple, everyday activities, such as sleeping, walking, watching television, and the like. With these recordings, a measure of total "uptime" can be obtained. "Uptime" is defined as the time the subject spends with his two feet on the floor. (Average daily uptime for a healthy person is around fifteen hours.) This can be used as an indicator of activity levels in the subject's own environment.

In an effort to use both the physical data that every physician traditionally employs in his diagnostic procedures and behavioral data collected from the patient in various paper-and-pencil tests, Steven F. Brena and Daniel L. Koch have proposed an operational definition of pain that can be clearly understood and communicated. This method, the Emory Pain Estimate Model, is designed to measure the severity of clinical pain by the analysis of three sets of data: (1) measures of tissue pathology (variations from normal findings in commonly used medical diagnostic tests, such as physical examination, neurologic examination, and radiologic and laboratory studies); (2) measures of pain behaviors (activity levels, pain verbalization, amount of drug intake, and personality-inventory test); (3) measures of the relationship between tissue pathology and behavior factors.

Data from the measurement of tissue pathology are coded on a linear horizontal scale of 0–10 points; similarly, measures of pain behaviors are depicted on a vertical scale of 0–10. The horizontal pathology scale is intersected midway by the vertical behavior scale to yield four quadrants, each representing a separate pain state or classification. Each classification describes a distinctly clinical profile and calls for different approaches to treatment. For instance, a Class I patient is a "pain-amplifier" who displays pain behavior in excess of demonstrable organic disease. Class I and Class III patients are pain-disabled and need behavior-modification therapy and functional reeducation. The Class IV patient is a "pain reducer" who displays minimal pain behavior in spite of considerable organic disease. Studies have shown that different raters looking over the same data agree on which quadrant patients should be placed in, suggesting that the method is quite reliable.

In another attempt to quantify clinical pain, Richard Black and Richard Chapman have defined each pain problem in terms of somatic (body) input, anxiety, and depression. They call their method the SAD Index, from the initials of the above terms. The magnitude of each component is computed from information derived from a series of clinical tests and psychological questionnaires, and is scaled along the axes of a three-dimensional system of rectangular coordinates. Each axis shows the magnitude of somatic inputs, anxiety factors, and depression problems on a scale of 0–10. The patient's total pain experience is then represented by the sum of the data scaled on the three axes.

Black and Chapman believe their SAD Index will enable a physician to assess pain problems in a more constructive way, looking at them as a composite of bodily, anxious, and depressive factors. This should result in a more meaningful clinical judgment, one that can be communicated more effectively to other health professionals.

A problem concerning the measurement of pain that has deep social and legal implications is related to cases where chronic-pain behavior is the major element in disability claims. In this area today, health professionals, insurance companies, industry, government, and legal professionals are up against a chaotic system. Few if any institutions provide a total approach to the evaluation of disabling chronic pain. Ideally, such an approach would not only measure pain, but would also provide a reliable impairment-and-disability rating, design a treatment program, and provide a specific judgment as to the patient's potential for returning to work.

As early as 1963, the American Medical Association laid out comprehensive guidelines for evaluation of disability as it relates to specific bodily systems. Unfortunately, the AMA method is quite complex and not altogether reliable. This is shown by the many cases in which two different physician-raters, using the same guidelines, have reached opposite conclusions.

The term "impairment" indicates a defect in the ability of the individual to function. It may be caused by a well-demonstrated disease process, but not necessarily. On the other hand, "disability" can involve a multitude of factors other than bodily dysfunction: motor performance, pain, motivation, fatigue, task performance, etc.

For instance, a person can have lung cancer but neither functional impairment nor disability to perform his job until the cancer has reached its terminal stage of growth, while a second individual, who happens to be a typist or violinist, can have a stiff little finger that considerably impairs the function of his hand and totally disables him for work.

In recent years, a fairly accurate and reliable disability-evaluation system known as the Hester System has been developed. This is a computerized method of measuring a person's vocational abilities. It consists of twenty-seven tests, such as motor performance, perceptual and intelligence tests, and reading and arithmetic abilities.

After testing, the raw scores are fed into a computer along with information about physical limitations, amount of possible training time, relationships with people, and working conditions to be avoided. The computer combines the best scores for all the categories and gives back information about jobs that best match the subject's characteristics.

Information gathered from the Hester Evaluation System is then integrated with data from medical evaluation, assessment of impairment based on AMA guidelines, and pain measurement and classification using one of the methods now available. This comprehensive system of disability seems to produce a fair, valid, and reliable judgment that is easy to communicate, because it is expressed in numerical values.

Consider the following example, using both the Emory Pain Estimate Model and the Hester Evaluation System to assess the case of a truck driver who complains of low-back pain and has filed for disability benefits after he suffers an on-the-job accident. The computer rating of his condition might read as follows:

Low-Back Pain, 32, M, P 1.5, B 8.5 Class I

Total Body Impairment 5%. Disability Rating 10%

In these numbers, a complete, sophisticated medical evaluation is summarized.

"32, M" simply identifies the patient as a thirty-two-year-old male.

"P 1.5" indicates a score of 1.5 on the pathology scale (minimal evidence of organic disease).

"B 8.5" on the behavior scale means a sick behavior is displayed far in excess of the pathologic rating, with evidence of drug abuse.

"Class I" points to a program of behavior modification as a treatment of choice.

Impairment rating of 5 percent and disability rating of 10 percent indicate the subject can perform almost every job. The computer printout will list "truck driver" among the jobs the subject can perform.

Studies at the Emory Pain Control Center have shown a significant relationship between chronic-pain states as classified by the Emory Pain Estimate Model and impairment/disability ratings. Out of 101 patients claiming disability for legal compensation, sixty-four were logged in Class I, with impairment ratings much lower than their disability scores. What this means is that over 50 percent of patients seeking compensation in accident cases showed pain behaviors in excess of evidence of organic disease. Their whole-body impairment was such that they could be vocationally trained to return to full productivity, if properly counseled.

When patients such as these are granted permanent disability benefits because of poor medical examinations, attorneys' gimmicks, and legal loopholes, they are likely to sink quickly into the misery of learned helplessness and swell the ranks of prematurely retired people. This points up the great importance of finding a way for professionals to agree on measurement techniques in chronic disabling-pain cases. Only by translating clinical judgments into numerical terms is it possible to reach reliable and valid conclusions in controversial cases.

The measurement of pain is like the work of a good detective case. In a thorough police investigation, all the facts are carefully gathered in a systematic way, weighed, and matched, then a conclusion is reached that points toward a suspect. In assessing pain in the absence of reliable physiological pain indicators, an accurate understanding of chronic pain can be reached only from a careful collection of pathologic, emotional, behavioral, and environmental data. By weighing and matching these facts, a clear picture of the whole problem emerges. The physician who tries to measure chronic pain on pathologic evidence only, the psychologist who looks at behavior only, the attorney whose only goal is to win a case in court—all of these serve the chronic sufferer poorly, even in cases where the sufferer himself seems to push the professional in a particular direction.

8

Comprehensive Treatment Programs for Chronic Pain States

S. F. BRENA

THE SLOW REALIZATION that pain is a multi-dimensional problem is bringing profound changes in the clinical approach to chronic pain. So-called pain-rehabilitation programs have multiplied in the United States in the last five years as evidence of this fact.

These programs seek to educate the sufferer to cope more effectively with his various physical and emotional problems. Basic goals common to all of them include: (1) detoxify the patient in case of drug abuse, using drug-withdrawal therapy; (2) desensitize him to sensory inputs that he has learned to perceive as painful; (3) train him scientifically to relax and perform some basic bracing exercises with a minimal expenditure of energy; (4) teach him to clearly discriminate between activity and pain, and between physical pain and emotional stress; (5) equip him with a coping behavior he can use in place of his old pain-drug behavior in times of stress.

Long-term results from pain-rehabilitation centers across the country are not yet available on a scale large enough to judge them accurately. The few reports so far published in medical journals seem to indicate that new hope is now available. However, most of the articles fail to show clearly what standards of measurement the success rates are based on, so a good statistical analysis can't be made.

It would be useful to analyze the emergence of the multidimensional attack on chronic pain in the framework of humankind's changing philosophy toward sickness and health over the ages.

The word "pain" is derived from both the Sanskrit *pu,* meaning "sacrifice," and the Latin word *poena,* meaning "punishment." These semantic roots of the English word "pain" clearly portray an idea of punishment in the pain experience, one that formed a part of our Judeo-Christian philosophy for thousands of years, until the present age. In the twentieth century, medicine sought to remove punishment from the pain condition, and for a while it promised freedom from pain to all human beings simply by killing germs, removing diseased organs, and balancing abnormal bodily functions, without asking the individual sufferer to make a personal effort to have a pain-free state of mind-body health. That effort has failed.

Medicine today is being forced by this failure to return to the ancient Hindu and Greek concepts of pain as a "holistic," or whole-person, experience involving body, mind, and spirit. This concept demands a personal commitment to a healthy lifestyle in a healthy environment as the basic requisite for freedom from pain.

The Greeks viewed pain as an experience born out of some failure in the right process of living. While aware of the brain and spinal cord, the Greeks did not understand how the nervous system functioned. Their thinking was based more on empirical observation and philosophical reasoning than on anatomic and physiological analysis.

Like the Egyptians before them, the Greeks attached greater importance to the heart than to the brain as a center where pain was perceived. For Aristotle, the heart was the site where all powers of the soul were manifested; to him, the changing motion of the heart accounted for most human feelings, including pain, which he defined as "a passion of the soul."

Alongside Greek logical thinking about medicine, a religious-medical cult grew up that became the most famous of its kind in history. This was the cult of Asclepius, whose first mention in Greek literature is found in Homer's *Iliad,* where Asclepius is represented as the father of all physicians, half-man, half-god. His cult gradually spread throughout Greece and was centered around temples known as *Asclepieia.* Here the patient would wait in silence and meditation for the transcendental experience of the god's visitation, which came during a sleep or trance. According to inscriptions, Asclepius cured paralysis, arthritic gout, headache, dyspepsia, epilepsy, and other chronic ailments.

The "Hymn for Asclepius" wirtten by the Greek dramatist Sophocles shows the great respect held by the Greeks for both the cult itself and for the *Asclepieia* "spa resorts." Many ancient rulers, including Alexander the Great,

Marcus Aurelius, and Julian were among the patients of *Asclepieia.* The very last words of Socrates dealt with Asclepius; on his deathbed the Greek philosopher instructed one of his disciples to pay an overdue bill to the healing god, as we read in the dialogue *Phaedo,* by Plato.

Greek medicine, while deeply rooted in a magic-religious background, also had many scientific, naturalistic, and speculative principles. The best known of these was the theory that all life processes are founded on the interplay of four basic elements: air, water, earth, and fire. In a healthy state the four energy-elements are balanced; disease comes when they are unbalanced. It was the job of the philosopher-physician to assist nature in the effort to keep the balance.

The idea of the four basic elements of life-energy actually originated in India, where it is well identified in the ancient writings known as the Vedas. From India the theory traveled westward; it was adopted and worked out by the Egyptians in the famous "Doctrine of Hermetes." It also went eastward and reappears in the Chinese conception of Yin and Yang, the two basic positive and negative life-forces. In Chinese folk-medicine, acupuncture is alleged to cure many painful ailments by reestablishing a state of balance between positive and negative life-forces.

In the West, the theory of the four life-energy elements went from Egypt to Greece. It survived the Roman Empire and the Middle Ages, reaching the modern age under the guise of new names and definitions. We know today from scientific research that all life processes are dependent on certain basic substances, with carbon among the most prominent, in various chemical combinations (earth). Oxygen (air) is necessary in most of our metabolic combustions (fire). We also know that living creatures contain more than half of their body weight in water. Definitions change, but basic life principles are recognized to be the same in all human cultures.

During the fifteen centuries between the fall of the Roman Empire and the modern age, Greek thought greatly influenced the development of Christian thinking. The art of medicine was still centered around the teachings of the great Greek philosophers; it continued to accept Aristotle's idea of pain as a "passion of the soul." Islamic philosopher-physicians such as Rhazes, Avicenna, Averroes, and Maimonides reflected the splendor of the Greek culture in the West's Dark Ages and made remarkable contributions to medical knowledge. To Rhazes we owe the first mention of "habits that become natural," which may be regarded as an early, though imperfect, sketch of conditioned behaviors.

There was no notion of pain as a neuro-anatomical phenomenon, however, For the Arabic physician, as well as for his Greek and European colleagues, pain remained a subjective, unfathomable "passion," with no acknowledged organic base. During the Renaissance, many discoveries about the anatomy of the brain, spinal cord, and sympathetic system were made and recorded in the monumental sixteenth-century work of Andreas Vesalius, *De humani corporis fabrica* (On the structure of the human body).

But Vesalius and other Renaissance scientists made little effort to give an anatomic and physiologic basis to the subjective experience of pain. Even René Descartes, in contrast to his attempt to fit the functioning of the human body into his mechanistic philosophy, denied that a nervous apparatus was involved in the pain experience. He continued to view pain as a "soul perception" located in the pineal gland and caused by an "excessive state of awareness."

From the early Hindu civilization (around 3000 B.C.) to the nineteenth century, the concept of pain and sickness as a state of life-energy unbalance—a sort of punishment for sinful living—dominated philosophical thought and related medical practice. Looked at in this way, the treatment of pain was more than a medical problem. It demanded that an individual commit himself to a changed lifestyle, to "repent" and "tune in" to spiritual and natural laws with medical and religious rituals.

The picture suddenly changed during the second half of the nineteenth century. When Louis Pasteur demonstrated that many diseases are caused by germs that reproduce within the body, a huge burden seemed lifted from the collective shoulders of men. Health no longer was a personal commitment to right thinking and right living but something to be negotiated with the legions of germs that could now be destroyed by chemical and immunologic warfare. Pain and sickness were no longer a "punishment" but something caused by nasty little creatures that attack us. Johannes Müller's theory of "specific nerve energy" fitted well with his changed attitude toward sickness and pain: to each specific germ the responsibility for each disease; to each specific nerve apparatus the task of transmitting each sensation to the brain, including the sense of pain.

As with almost every field of knowledge at the turn of the last century, the application of the principles of experimental science made metaphysical and philosophical doctrines obsolete. New hopes were raised, that by properly understanding and manipulating physical phenomena, a solution could be found for all health problems, including the dreadful specter of pain.

Between the time of Louis Pasteur (1822–1895) and the second half of the twentieth century, a span of about a hundred years, more progress in medical knowledge and related therapeutic skills and technology was achieved than during the preceding three thousand years. The battle against infectious diseases was brilliantly won. Once-deadly diseases such as diabetes and other metabolic disorders now have low mortality rates; their victims have a fair chance of normal living. Has pain been conquered? Acute pain certainly has been subdued and the dreadful agony of surgical and traumatic injuries suffered without any analgesia has largely faded from the memory of mankind. But the struggle against chronic pain is still going on. No easy solution is available now and one is not likely to be found in the foreseeable future.

Between the late 1920s and early 1960s, hope was high that chronic pain might be controlled by surgical or chemical interruption of the nervous system's pain-pathways. However, as noted earlier, recent studies have shown that there is more than one system involved in the transmission of pain impulses. Surgery for chronic pain has produced disappointingly low rates of success, with a grave danger of actually increasing the pain experience through destruction of nerve fibers.

In 1955 two neurosurgeons, J. C. White and W. H. Sweet, wrote an optimistic book about the control of chronic pain by neurosurgery. In 1969 the same two authors wrote another book in which they reexamined their own long-term results in relief of pain by surgical interruption of nervous pathways. They candidly recognized the limitations, dangers, and poor results of this type of surgery, and wisely cautioned against indiscriminate use of such procedures.

Current medical literature reveals a frustrating sense of

confusion in regard to hard-to-prove theories about the neurophysiology of pain. There are contrasting and disappointing results from almost every therapy aimed at relieving chronic pain.

Meanwhile, it is becoming clear that if indeed there are nerve pathways that transmit pain impulses, these systems are under the control of a multitude of emotional and cognitive factors that profoundly affect the pain experience itself. Like the ancient Hindu and Greek philosophers, the modern scientist must admit that the phenomenon of pain is more than a simple pathologic problem, such as a gunshot wound or arthritis. It is a holistic experience involving the individual in his totality, with deep roots in his environment.

9

Emotions and Pain

W. H. BIGGERS

WHEN NORMAN P. FELL AT WORK and broke his arm, he was able to deal appropriately with his pain and injury. A physician reduced the fracture and applied a cast; Norman then returned to his job with some disability. His discomfort, however, was not great. His fellow workers and supervisors took note of his injury and gave him adequate emotional support until the process of healing was complete. He was soon back to full function.

Sometime later, when Allen M., one of Norman's coworkers, fell and suffered a similar blow on his arm, there was no discernible injury. Even the most extensive medical examination failed to reveal a fracture, a sprain, or harm to a peripheral nerve. The fall did, in fact, cause a brief period of discomfort that led Allen to believe he had been seriously injured. But lack of medical evidence of injury compelled him to return to his job. Allen, less emotionally stable and less tolerant of physical injuries than Norman, goes back to work, but with the conviction that he has a yet undiagnosed injury.

Allen's peers now treat him as though nothing had happened. Unlike Norman, he wears no cast. He is perplexed and embarrassed. He really *feels* pain in his arm. He is not deliberately misrepresenting its presence (malingering). As Allen talks about his pain to others, attempting to explain its presence, his painful experience consciously and unconsciously intensifies. Allen begins to work less efficiently than Norman, whose arm is still in a cast. Eventually he begins a long series of consultations with various physicians, trying to find someone in authority who will confirm his feeling of pain.

As we noted earlier, man is different from animals in his ability to translate an emotional response to his environment into something he identifies as *somatic* or bodily pain. Psychologically, the translation of an emotional feeling such as anxiety or depression into pain is called somatization. In the example just cited, Allen has *somatized* his imagined injury and feelings of anxiety into a case of chronic pain.

Pain feelings of this type can be understood by anyone who has a headache brought on by tension. We are able to deal with the headache in a reasonable way, and do not assume it is caused by a serious disorder inside our heads. Indeed, many times we are able to identify the stress at home or at work that triggers the physiologic and anatomic events that cause the headache. The headache disappears spontaneously or responds to mild analgesics, and we think no more of it.

Unfortunately, Allen identifies nothing beyond the fact

he has fallen and struck his arm, and now his arm hurts. He makes no connection with other events in his life. He does not connect his aching arm with the conflict he is having with his supervisors, or with the fact that he feels inadequate when comparing himself with his peers and clumsy in allowing himself to fall. He might have been better served by a tangible injury that would have gained him concern and support. Lacking this, he magnifies, misinterprets, and distorts his feelings in a way that does secure what his emotions tell him he needs—the concern of others.

Allen experiences frustration, anxiety, anger, and depression. He is now governed by the somatization of his feelings, which he describes to anyone who will listen as "excruciating" pain in his arm. Eventually, he regresses to an infantile level of behavior that has nothing to do with true cause-and-effect. Such behavior does, however, allow him to think of his situation as realistic without admitting that it draws on infantile rather than mature behavioral patterns.

When events have progressed this far, intervention must take place at several levels. Allen must come to some understanding of the sequence of events that has brought him here. He must be helped to reconstruct these events in such a way that they become understandable to him in terms of emotional pain rather than physical pain. This distinction is essential, and without its acceptance by the pain victim, very little can be done to alleviate the condition. Once the distinction is made, medication can be given for Allen's specific emotional state. Psychotherapy can also begin to help him cope with his emotions in the future.

The chronic-pain sufferer has two choices: He can either

subconsciously deal with his problems in a way that creates a feeling of high self-esteem and addresses itself to the real cause of his feelings, or he can subconsciously deal with them in a hysterical and unrealistic fashion.

George Engel has shown that pain is sometimes related to guilt feelings that the patient has failed to identify correctly. In his work with ulcerative colitis patients, he noted that headaches were the most common symptom felt by such patients when they were not actually experiencing periods of greatly increased trouble with their colons. He concluded that headaches were an alternate symptom that occurred in these patients when they were feeling intense guilt, either consciously or unconsciously, after they made an important decision, took an extremely active stand on an important issue, or felt themselves to be uncommonly in control of their feelings.

In these situations, the patients did not have feelings of helplessness or fear, and this was in dramatic contrast with the unassertive, passive, and helpless attitudes they usually felt prior to an attack of colitis. Headaches during an episode of colitis often came just before the end of the attack. Engel believed that the dissipation of guilt feelings in the colitis patients by way of headaches was related both to the prevention of an attack of their illness and to the ending of actual attacks. Accepting Engel's premise, we can take this as another example of people reacting physically to their feelings; if such feelings are allowed to be expressed in some appropriate fashion, the illness is greatly modified and often relieved.

Another problem that involves the translation of an emotional insult into physical pain is seen in the condition known as conversion hysteria. In this situation, the individual may have a symptom such as loss of capacity to move an arm or leg, or he may manifest his imbalanced emotions with chronic pain complaints. In some patients, both paralysis and pain are present.

An example of conversion hysteria occurred in the case of Alice W., a young woman who worked in a textile mill. Renovation work was being done around her work area and a large overhead air-conditioning unit had been set in place but not secured in its brackets. As she worked at her sewing machine, the unit slipped free of its brackets and fell, grazing her right arm. Had it fallen six inches more to the right, it would have crushed her arm; twelve inches closer and it might have killed her.

The young woman's anxiety over this event was overwhelming; her co-workers escorted her to an anteroom where she could calm down and rest. After about thirty minutes, she felt better and decided to return to work. At this point, however, she found herself completely unable to move her right arm. She began to notice an increasing amount of discomfort in the arm. This gradually became more intense until she was forced to go home, and she was thereafter unable to return to her job.

A medical evaluation failed to uncover a reason for the paralysis or the pain. To the frustration of both Alice and the physician, nothing could be done about it. Since there was no injury, it seemed reasonable that there could be neither paralysis nor pain; there was no way of treating something that could not exist. All witnesses agreed that the events had occurred as described. Alice herself was the first to categorically state that she had been barely touched by the falling equipment and was not injured by it. However, the fact remained that the symptoms were connected with the falling of the air-conditioning unit, and that her pain and paralysis continued, fixed and unrelenting.

Alice went to a psychiatrist and told the same story. It

was decided that she should be made more aware of her actual feelings at the time of the initial insult. In this way she might help herself and her physician by revealing what her feelings had been.

Under hypnosis, Alice recalled her fear of having come close to serious injury or death. She also indicated that her fear had been so intense she felt unable to reenter the same situation that had almost killed her. It was clear that the pain and paralysis had resulted from an unconscious translation of intense emotional feelings into physical symptoms that effectively prevented her from returning to the same life-threatening situation. There followed a number of sessions under hypnosis in which Alice talked about her anxiety. She was encouraged to reduce her intense feelings of fear, and it was suggested to her in the hypnotic state that no harm would befall her by allowing the return of function and remission of pain in her right arm. Gradually she recognized her initial fear and her fantasy that it would happen again with fatal results: She realized that she possessed more effective ways of dealing with the situation. Alice recovered to the point where she was able to ask her supervisor for a different type of job in another area of the factory. Her anxiety abated along with her symptoms, which she no longer needed to protect her from what she had perceived as a dangerous situation.

As in somatization, hysterical symptoms are unconscious. They do serve a function, perhaps a questionable one, by allowing the individual to cope with his total environment. Unfortunately, this coping mechanism does not allow the person to adapt properly to the real-life situation that causes the stress, and in the final analysis, it is a poor way to adapt to one's problems.

Another difficult problem for both the patient and his physician involves organic disorders that do not relate to the subjective pain-experience as it is described by the patient. Bob B., for instance, was wounded in the leg in Vietnam, but today the pain manifests itself by an excruciating burning sensation in his right shoulder, a condition that keeps Bob from resuming his former trade as a bricklayer.

In pain cases that defy a reasonable explanation based on the extent or location of the organic lesion, it is clear that the services of professionals who can deal directly with the physical pain as well as others who can treat the emotional overlay are required. Without this kind of joint effort, therapy is seldom complete or satisfactory. In a joint approach, the two different professional disciplines enhance each other and usually achieve a more favorable result.

By treating the organic problem with drugs or physical intervention and by relieving the psychic elements simultaneously, each component of the total pain is given some relief. Most physical diseases involve an emotional reaction that makes the patient more aware of his pain and sensitizes him to it. Treating the physical component while ignoring the psychological element can be compared with removing an appendix without bothering to suture the wound. Management of pain is not complete without considering the psychological components, whether they were present before the physical injury occurred or came as a result of the injury.

People who are emotionally healthy prefer to deal directly with emotional problems. This is the best way for them to resolve issues and to continue normal functioning. When a person's defense mechanisms fail, he may experience emotional discomfort without addressing himself to the real issues. He may allow himself to stay marginally stable from an emotional point of view, but he will be largely dysfunctional.

If we resort to our more primitive or infantile defenses against daily challenges, we tend to lose the connection between a trauma and our reaction to it, such as the feeling of pain. Trying to recapture the cause and effect some months later is a much more formidable task than dealing with the problem initially.

In terms of chronic pain, the vulnerability of a person who suffers from low self-esteem or lack of self-worth is increased many-fold. Confronted by emotional stress, he will almost inevitably resort to a concrete expression of his distress; not uncommonly, he will express it as physical pain. This reaction must not be dismissed as a conscious falsification of symptoms. Rather, it shows that the individual has a serious problem in dealing with reality.

10

A New Medical Specialist: The Algologist, or "Pain Expert"

S. F. BRENA

AT THIS POINT it may be of interest to trace briefly the evolution of the concept of chronic pain within the medical profession. Then we will depict the essential roles to be played by pain-control centers and by a new kind of community physician, the algologist, in grappling with the problem of chronic pain today.

René Leriche was probably the first twentieth-century physician to recognize chronic pain as a particular disease-state different from other diseases. In his book *The Surgery of Pain,* published after World War I, Leriche made original observations on a number of painful disorders that seem to feed on themselves, with increasing subjective pain and no clear sign of growing damage to organ systems.

To Leriche we owe many ideas and pioneering techniques for dealing with chronic pain. Some of his methods are still popular today; among them is the use of a procedure called sympathectomy for the painful condition known as causalgia, a syndrome of burning, excruciating pain that may develop after gunshot wounds. Sympathectomy involves a severance of certain ganglia in the sympathetic nervous system. (While Leriche was the first to perform surgery for causalgia, it was an American physician, Weir Mitchell, who gave us the first vivid and detailed description of this painful disorder, which he repeatedly observed in soldiers wounded during the War between the States.)

We owe to an Italian-born American, John J. Bonica, the first lucid, systematic approach to the pain-disease concept. In 1953, Bonica published his monumental work *The Management of Pain.* In this now-classic textbook, Bonica laid down a clear picture of what pain is and how it should be diagnosed and managed. Most of the chapters in his book are still valid, even though written twenty-five years ago, when the neurological and behavioral sciences were still relatively primitive in knowledge of pain.

I consider myself fortunate in having been a student of both Leriche and Bonica: in 1948, during my year of internship at the American Hospital in Paris, and in 1956, when I took a fellowship in Bonica's department, then based at Tacoma (Washington) General Hospital.

A highlight in development of the pain-disease concept was the publication in 1965 by Ronald Melzack and Patrick Wall of their "gate-control" theory, which brought together much of the scattered knowledge about the human nervous system and opened the way for new research into the mechanisms by which certain impulses from the periphery of the body are translated into subjective painful feelings.

As a logical consequence of the gate-control theory, techniques of electrical nerve stimulation for suppression of pain were quickly developed and became clinically known in the late 1960s, when Norman Shealy and others announced their findings on the electrical inhibition of pain by stimulation of the dorsal (back) section of the spinal cord. Later, the technique of dorsal-column stimulation, which requires the implantation of electrodes in the spinal cord, was abandoned in favor of the easier and equally effective technique of transcutaneous (outside-the-skin) electrical nerve stimulation. These methods will be described in more detail in a later chapter.

Another revolutionary technique was proposed and demonstrated in the early 1960s by John Basmajian and a few others; it showed that "motor units" in the muscles, as well as functions of the autonomic nervous system, can be brought under control of the mind and will by learning techniques. The ground was thus set for biofeedback training.

Another important stage in the evolution of pain treatment closely followed the pioneering work by Wilbert Fordyce and his colleagues on the involvement of learning in problems of chronic pain. Once the learning process was shown to play a role in chronic pain, one of its mysteries was solved: A scientific reason was given for the paradox of habitual sufferers having little evidence of organic disease. "Learned pain" became a useful model on which research projects and treatment programs were based.

So an idea born between the two World Wars reached its climax in the past decade, when it was demonstrated scientifically that chronic pain involved nervous mechanisms different from those that influence acute pain. Research proved that learning processes deeply influence the pain experience; it was also shown that we can learn to control our pain feelings.

Despite all this, the new knowledge about chronic pain has not been widely adopted by physicians in general medical practice; even more so, it has remained largely ignored by legal professionals and legislators.

Problems of chronic pain are best approached by teams of highly specialized professionals from various health disciplines who share the knowledge, skill, and motivation to deal with this illness. This concept of multidisciplinary teamwork, first proposed by John Bonica, has stimulated much new thinking, new technology for treatment, and new research. So far, however, it has failed to break through its restricted circle of "experts" and motivate clinical practitioners or young medical doctors to devote their professional skills to the diagnosis and treatment of chronic-pain disorders.

In 1956, when I was a resident physician at the Tacoma General Hospital Pain Clinic, there were few pain-control facilities in the United States or abroad. In 1976 a report published in the magazine *Medical World News* listed only seventeen pain clinics and pain-control centers in the United States, most of them based at universities in large metropolitan areas.

The American Association of Anesthesiologists is compiling an updated directory of pain-control centers in this country. This new directory will probably show a few more pain clinics than in the 1976 listing. By and large, however, the total number of pain clinics is far too small for our huge population of chronic sufferers, many of whom are disabled by a lifestyle governed by pain and drugs.

Many of the world's "pain experts" met in Seattle, Washington, in 1973, at an International Symposium on Pain, and began an attack on this problem. They agreed on the urgent need to stimulate interest in chronic pain among young doctors. In consequence, the International Association for the Study of Pain (IASP) was founded and incorporated in 1974.

An impressive surge of interest in pain problems followed this move; the first congress of the IASP, held in Florence, Italy, in 1975, was attended by over 1,100 registrants from thirty-five countries and seventy-five different health disciplines. It was the largest meeting ever held of professionals with a common interest in pain issues. A pain-clinic movement has been triggered by the founding of the IASP and is gaining momentum. Focus on chronic pain has sharpened in the health-delivery system and particularly in the medical profession. Continuing medical education courses and conferences, audio-visual programs, and regional and national symposia on pain problems have multiplied during the last few years; there has been excellent attendance by health professionals and good press coverage. From all these activities, a new concept is emerging.

But it is my opinion that the problem of chronic pain, with its many interconnected factors, won't be solved unless professional assistance for chronic sufferers is widely applied where the suffering people live—in their own communities—and not in university centers alone. This can't be done unless physicians trained in this field are ready to take up the challenge and go where the sufferers are.

A new kind of medical practice is called for: algology, the science of pain assessment and control. Algology is derived from two Greek words, *algos* ("pain") and *logos* ("discipline" or "study"). The need for such a discipline has been acknowledged and a branch of the IASP has been organized as an American Pain Association to promote the science of algology and possibly set criteria for its certification and recognition.

The future directions of algology are open for discussion and will certainly be controversial. In calling myself an algologist, I think of a person in this discipline as a physician with average medical expertise—comparable with that of a general practitioner—plus a good background in the neurosciences and advanced training in rehabilitation medicine, behavioral medicine, and current treatment methods for pain. Such a practice can be helpful both to chronic sufferers and the community at large. In addition to delivering comprehensive health care in cases of chronic pain, the local algologist-physician can disseminate information among his peers and to the general public. He can help settle long-standing cases of pain-related disability and lend a part of his professional time to assisting the legal community in better understanding the issues involved in disabling-pain problems.

The algologist can promote the collection of epidemiological data on pain as a disease state—data urgently needed by those who cry out for changes in our social approaches to the pain-disease state. The algologist can act as a consultant to various agencies concerned with the social and financial assistance of the chronically sick patient. He or she can generate momentum for lawmaking bodies to review disability and sickness-compensation laws that may no longer be responsive to our changed knowledge of pain.

Can chronic pain be brought under control by the installation of pain-study and research centers staffed by competent algologists throughout the country? Figures on this subject are lacking and the few we have are far from conclusive. But one report, prepared by the New England Rehabilitation Hospital's Pain Unit in Woburn, Massachusetts, indicates promising results, and a reduction in the "doctor-shopping" and other "pain games" usually seen in chronic pain victims. The study concerns twenty-five in-patients admitted to the hospital for chronic-pain problems between January 1975 and June 1976, with follow-up times ranging up to twelve months. Some of the results of the study:

1. Average duration of illness before treatment: 56.8 months per patient.
2. Days of hospitalization after rehabilitation treatment: a 73 percent decrease.
3. Hospital admissions after treatment: a 56 percent decrease.
4. Cost before treatment: $2,987 per-patient per-year average. Cost after treatment: $820 per-patient per-year average. (These figures do not include the gains of returning to work with conversion of dependence into independence.)
5. No surgical procedure for chronic pain was performed after patients went into rehabilitation program.

A random survey of 100 patients examined at the Emory Pain Control Center was taken in 1978 in order to assess the effectiveness of treatment in educating chronic sufferers to be more active, with less reliance on drugs for support. Most of these patients had chronic back pain of many years duration and had seen many physicians with little relief from their discomfort and no return to normal functioning. Results after completion of the six-week out-patient pain-control program show:

1. *Performance levels:* average increase from 3 hours 45 minutes to 6 hours 11 minutes of diversified physical activities.

2. *Drug intake for pain.* The number of patients taking narcotics decreased from 60 to 5; the number of patients taking tranquilizers decreased from 44 to 1. At the onset of treatment, most of these patients feared that increasing physical activities and reducing reliance on drugs would increase their discomfort; the opposite proved true.

3. *Changes in subjective pain experience.* Using the McGill Pain Questionnaire, patients recorded a reduction in pain intensity from 72% before treatment to 53% after treatment, average.

Checks of follow-up results showed continued maintenance of improvement in performance levels, drug use, and pain-intensity ratings several months after treatment.

There are many reasons why pain-control units staffed by algologist-physicians can treat chronic pain more effectively and yet less expensively:

1. All features of treatment are done in one place at one time, thus reducing the patient's time off the job, travel expenses, etc.

2. Rehabilitation techniques are noninvasive, or at least much less invasive and less expensive than surgical procedures; most are done without hospitalization.

3. When hospitalization is needed, it requires lim-

ited nursing services and no expense for acute medical care, such as recovery room or intensive-care units.

4. Multiple medical workups are kept down by a comprehensive approach to the patient's health problems.

5. Disability cases can be settled promptly when a computerized disability-evaluation system is associated with a pain-control unit.

6. In a community with a pain clinic, public information about pain is likely to be better. As a result, chronic sufferers from a large referral area can opt for treatment other than drugs and surgery, with a related decrease in morbidity and disability.

7. Experience at the Emory Pain Control Center has shown that when a trained group of algologists provides services in cases involving pending disability claims, communication is improved between health and legal professionals. The result is a reduction in the number of long-standing cases in litigation for disability benefits, and an increase in the efficiency of pain measurement and counseling.

11

Toward a Pain-Free Society

S. F. BRENA

IN MANY WAYS, we can look on chronic pain in its disabling form as an admission of failure. On physiological grounds, it is a failure of the brain's intelligent power to exercise control when a disease strikes and sets in motion pain-producing impulses. From an emotional perspective, it is a failure to recognize and deal realistically with negative feelings; we convert them instead into maladaptive behaviors. From an existential point of view, it is a failure to meet challenges and to live up to our dignity as human beings; we escape instead into the dubious refuge of tranquilizers, sleeping pills, and helplessness. On a spiritual level, it is a failure to surrender to a greater dimension of love and selflessness.

But chronic, disabling pain is not only an admission of

failure for the individual. To a greater degree, it is also a failure of the medical profession, which still insists on treating chronic pain as a mere symptom of disease, something to be "cured" by cutting it out of the body or drugging it out of the mind. Too many unnecessary operations; a too-liberal prescription policy with drugs of doubtful value; too many hospitalizations for pain complaints; too many useless, duplicating, expensive medical workups for chronic pain of long duration—all these things actually teach patients new repertoires in their conditioned sick-behaviors while wrecking their finances and emotional stability.

Finally, chronic pain is an admission of our society's failure to deal with this particular human problem more intelligently. Our social emphasis is on health, but health is viewed as a gift to be begged for, one involving medical manipulations and drug prescriptions. Instead, health should be a right we earn by our personal commitment to healthy and ethical living. The concept of human wholeness is still lacking in our social approach to health care; the appeal is not to the individual to grow in health consciousness, but to the taxpayer to provide more funds to support more agencies to teach the unfortunate sufferer to become even more helpless, depressed, nonproductive, and unhappy.

Let a person be sick or injured, and enormous pressure is brought on him to perpetuate his sick role and maintain his dependency on others. If the injury has legal implications, attorneys and claims adjusters join physicians and family members in the senseless task of keeping the injured person dependent, withdrawn, angrily unhappy, and maladjusted.

I have sat through so many legal depositions that I have few doubts about the sickness-reinforcing roles played by legal professionals in claims for damages in cases of disabling chronic illness. I have infuriated more than one attorney by telling them, "You may win your legal case by pressing a questionable issue of sickness, but you will almost certainly contribute to keeping your client in a condition of emotional illness and learned helplessness."

This melancholy state of affairs is readily seen in our current laws providing compensation for on-the-job injuries. The injured worker is paid disability benefits for as long as he claims sickness and inability to work, then his benefits are promptly reduced and eventually abolished as soon as he returns to work. These laws require the employer to take upon himself (and pass on to his customers) the risk of accepting an injured employee back on his job—an employee who initially may not be as efficient as he was before the accident.

Certainly, such an employee needs a great deal of emotional and technical support before he is able to resume full work-productivity. Under the fundamental law of effect that underlies the major principles of learning and performance (people do things that pay off), the present laws for workmen's compensation are a perfect example of rewarding sick behaviors and guaranteeing that management will be reticent about helping injured workers return to their old positions.

The psychological impact of any disabling illness is enormous. In an attempt to cope with his problem, the sufferer goes through sequences of defense mechanisms, such as denial of the problem, withdrawal, somatization, regression into a childlike state of dependency, and maladaptive rationalization accompanied by anger and hostility. If the injured person is properly helped, he may quickly reach a point of acceptance. He can then start building a new self-image that will permit him to adopt work behaviors better adapted to his changed lifestyle following an injury or disease. His physiological needs and his quest for economic security and love must be met with a structured program designed to promote healthy roles and play down illness-behaviors.

It would be much more sensible to take some of the money from the huge sums currently paid to maintain workers in a state of conditioned sickness and use it to provide economic incentives for the injured worker, encouraging him to return to work as soon as the acute phase of the injury is over and the attending physician has released him for return to productive activities. It would also seem logical to obtain the cooperation of employers in rehiring employees as soon as they have recovered, perhaps at different duties, by granting such employers tax rebates for every worker rehired. Again, it would be far more ethical to give proper recognition to professionals who show proficiency in handling workmen's compensation cases, and who are successful in reeducating injured workers, so that they will promptly return to work.

In the Introduction, John Bonica advocates a massive "crash" program to deal with the enormous problem of chronic pain in moving toward a relatively pain-free society. Such a program, in our view, should be centered around several pivotal targets:

1. *Research.* Our knowledge of pain is still imperfect and must be expanded with a great deal of new and sophisticated research. Public and private funds should go into such research areas as:

(*a*) *Neurophysiology of pain.* As scientists probe deeper into the mysteries of the nervous system, they discover more questions than answers as to how the impulses that carry information about bodily damage become the perception of pain: The role of brain mechanisms in filtering and controlling pain-producing impulses is far from clear; the balance systems between nerve activity, hormones, and body chemistry are largely uncharted; and so on.

(*b*) *Pharmacology of pain.* The discovery of opiate receptors in certain brain areas and of chemicals manufactured by the body with effects similar to those of morphine—endomorphin or enkephalin—has opened new horizons of thinking and research. Pharmacologists already are speaking of chronic pain as "a syndrome of deficiency in endomorphin/enkephalin." In their speculations, certain forms of chronic pain are roughly compared with diabetes, a disease of insulin deficiency. In other words, the bodies of certain individuals may lack something in the production of endomorphin and are thus more exposed to painful perceptions when a disease or injury strikes. The far-reaching implications of this speculation are worth all the cost of further scientific investigation.

(*c*) *Epidemiology of pain.* Chronic pain is probably the number one health problem in the United States, as indicated by Bonica in the Introduction. Yet, epidemiological information—information gathered on the characteristic features of a disease process—on this problem is largely unavailable, and urgently needed, if action is to be taken to curb the cost of chronic pain and suffering.

(*d*) *Psychology of pain.* The relationship between personality and chronic pain, our ability to learn chronic pain and sickness, the role of helplessness and hopelessness in reinforcing the pain experience, the impact of social and cultural factors—these are only a few of many areas in which our knowledge is primitive and needs clarification.

(*e*) *Classification and measurement of pain.* An entire chapter has been written on this subject; its importance in a comprehensive pain-study program cannot be overemphasized. Although countless textbooks on pain are available, they present the pain phenomenon in a bewildering variety of perspectives, each according to the author's own experience and field of knowledge. The result is an enormous confusion in terminology and definitions, starting with the cornerstone definition of acute versus chronic pain. This semantic confusion taxes communication among professionals heavily. It must be cleared away to allow greater cross-fertilization of knowledge among doctors and between doctors and laymen.

2. *Public information about pain and health.* If freedom from pain is to be achieved through personal commitments to health, public information is crucial. Preventive medicine and the communications media have done excellent work in giving the public information about health and disease. Such TV programs usually aren't run in prime viewing time, however, and the management of TV stations is usually reluctant to wade into controversial issues. Health programs are like fireside chats among gentlemen in the same club. Presented in this way, health information lacks sufficient clout to make an impact on general audiences.

We can speculate on what might happen if an information campaign dealing with chronic pain, chronic sickness, and drug abuse related to these problems were mounted in prime TV-time in the style of an all-out effort to sell a commercial product. What would be the effects of showing pictures of lungs ravished by smoking, or livers destroyed by heavy drinking? What impact would there be with no-holds-barred stories of people who made themselves chronically ill with unhealthy lifestyles? Why shouldn't honesty and fairness demand that for every drug advertised in public media, its side effects must also be mentioned as part of the same message? We should apply the "feedback" principle to public information programs about health and disease: Let people know and see for themselves the consequences of their own habits, so that corrections can be made, if necessary.

3. *Involvement of lawmakers and legal professionals in a massive study of pain.* Because chronic pain, among other things, is an "ecological" disease with deep roots in the social and legal bedrock of our culture, the cooperation of lawmakers and the legal fraternity is essential if we are to have a pain-free society.

Thirty-three percent of all patients seen at the Emory Pain Control Center for chronic pain are workmen's compensation cases; the pain problem has been triggered by an accident on the job. Another 18% of the chronic sufferers have other pending legal claims, mostly for traffic accidents.

These figures indicate that in 51% of the cases examined at the Emory Pain Control Center, the findings of the physicians are at some point cross-examined by attorneys and are possibly influential in determining a judicial ruling. How poorly these two different groups of professionals communicate, can only be inferred by the fact that physicians and attorneys speak completely different languages and provide service under different codes of ethics.

The physician is consulted for obtaining relief of pain, but the attorney is hired to win the litigation and to obtain compensation. In court, pain behaviors must be emphasized, whereas—often at the same time—the physician is trying hard to control them. The result is often an emotional chaos for the chronic sufferer caught between two different situations with no control over either of them.

Efforts, therefore, should be made by medical and legal professional associations to organize educational courses where doctors and attorneys can meet, discuss their common problems, and learn to improve their mutual understanding and communication.

Research in pain must be followed by social and legislative action to translate scientific findings into practical rules and laws. One recent, hopeful example of such cooperation has been the impact that research into the dangers of smoking has had in producing laws and regulations designed to inform and protect the public.

One delicate area of concern is how far we can go in translating human compassion into laws. We've emphasized the miscarriage of our compassionate laws relating to disability, which actually foster and perpetuate conditions of unproductivity and misery in large numbers of people. How far should a society go in protecting the individual against himself? Is it ethical to ask taxpayers to shoulder indefinitely the burden of disability claims for people who've hurt themselves by reckless, drunken driving; by being shot in tavern brawls; by overeating, oversmoking, and overdrinking in spite of being warned?

By granting easy access to a lifestyle of paid disability through Social Security, aren't we inviting emotionally weak people to act irresponsibly toward themselves and others, knowing that society will protect them if they get hurt? Is it fair to overload and put into near-bankruptcy a Social Security system designed to protect the dignity and welfare of senior citizens by picking up the tab for chronic pain in cases that involve irresponsible social behavior? These are just a few of the many questions that a national study of pain might answer and submit for consideration to political leaders and legislators.

The present legal definition of "disability" is medically incorrect and financially irresponsible. It assumes that a 26-year-old worker who is unable to work because of a mild injury suffered on the job, by law should be given the same disability benefits as a 58-year-old man who cannot work because of cancer. The latter is probably beyond reasonable hope of recovery, but the young man can be promptly returned to gainful employment as soon as his injury has healed. Instead, he is told that he is disabled indefinitely, and he is given compensation for remaining in artificial idleness.

Moreover, because it is based on an incorrect definition, the present legislation on disability is unfair. It rewards with compensation not always the true sufferer, but more often the expert in "painmanship," the person who is proficient at the "pain game" and capable of convincing physicians, attorneys, and administrative law judges that he is truly in "excruciating pain," "cannot go to work because of his pain," and therefore deserves disability benefits.

New legislation is before Congress that would reform the Social Security disability program in a manner that would make the program more humanitarian, while at the same time reducing its escalating costs. Among the principal features of one such bill (H.R. 5064) is a new definition of disability that would replace the current system's tendency to sentence a person who is disabled to a lifetime of helplessness and nonproductivity. A witness for this bill last year told the Subcommittee on Social Security of the House Committee on Ways and Means, "The present law is creating drones rather than workers."

By establishing a termination date as well as a beginning date for all disability benefits, except for the "hard core" disabled, the proposed law would encourage beneficiaries of Social Security disability payments to return to work. The Society of Actuaries has estimated that if such a definition had been enacted in 1975, the program costs in 1977 would have been reduced by more than $2 billion.

A second aspect of the bill would save additional billions of dollars by requiring a 100 percent review of all cases, thus helping to remove unqualified recipients from the program. The new legislation would also establish equality under the law; it would reduce the number of appeals and require the disability-insurance trust fund to be defended at the initial stages of the legal process. It was estimated that just one successful defense of the trust fund would save over $56,000.

4. *Changes in the philosophy of medical science.* While preventive medicine is a well-established and active

branch of medicine, there is no question that the practice of medicine is heavily oriented toward curing or controlling rather than preventing the disease process. Knowing that the health industry ranks among the leading business endeavors in the United States, it is sad to report that such a vital industry operates, on the whole, like an automobile business that is willing to do repair work but shows little concern for preventive maintenance. It may be quite reluctant, in fact, to take the time to give a lot of frank and open information to customers on the subject of prevention.

As everyone knows, failure in preventive maintenance often cripples a car and stalls it on the highway after a few thousand miles. In a similar fashion, the lack of preventive medical maintenance can speed up the aging process and expose the individual to early, unnecessary pain and physical disability.

The impact of the mind on the body, along with techniques of training mind-power to control bodily functions, are still poorly understood and primitive in design. They are thus largely ignored by a majority of physicians, although this area holds bright promise for the future and should be carefully studied by every health professional involved in chronic pain.

The field of rehabilitation is a third area in which medicine has yet to realize its full potential. A number of studies, all with similar results, have shown that the level of independent function on admission to rehabilitation is about 35 percent of normal for stroke, spinal-cord injury, arthritis, and amputation patients combined. At discharge, however, function has risen to 70 percent of normal; and at follow-up two to three years later, it is up to about 75 percent of normal.

It is estimated that the lifetime savings for a single patient following rehabilitation for acute spinal cord injury is nearly $60,000; this includes both increased earnings and decreased costs of medical and nursing care. "For the five thousand Americans with new spinal-cord injuries in one year, this represents a national lifetime net savings of $300 million just for careful rehabilitation of *one type* of catastrophic injury," says J. Robin deAndrade, director of the Center for Rehabilitation Medicine at Emory University. "Nothing at all has been said about what independence and ability to work means to an individual who has been severely disabled, and to his or her family," Dr. deAndrade adds. "The returned opportunity for life, liberty, and the pursuit of happiness is priceless."

In this regard, there is abundant evidence that people who are happy and satisfied in their work live longer than those who are not. In the Soviet Union, a study of the Abkhasian people revealed that 2.5 percent were ninety years or older, compared with 0.1 percent of all Russians, and 0.4 percent of Americans. Among the Abkhasian people, lifelong work is a distinguishing factor; even those who are one hundred or older put in as much as four hours a day on their farms.

The United States system encourages nonwork among the chronically ill and elderly. Many older Americans who are otherwise healthy adopt a "sick role" that gains them admittance to a nursing home. Often they do this because they are rejected by their families. Instead of sanctioning among our elderly a sick role that encourages excessive use of the health-care system and psychosomatic complaints, wouldn't it be more humane to make it possible for older citizens to continue working, with increasing prestige in their later years, as do the Abkhasian and a few other societies?

Quite properly, medical science has been slow to accept change without challenge. But profound changes are mandatory if medicine is to deal with the consequences of its own triumphs in prolonging the lives of people who would otherwise have died. Even a wealthy society such as ours can't afford indefinitely to foot the bill of keeping alive but unproductive the millions who've survived once-deadly diseases such as chronic heart and kidney diseases. Medicine must meet this looming crisis with ingenuity and imagination, not regression; it must take the lead in educating and informing the public and in creating an environment conducive to personal health-maintenance by all Americans.

The emergence of algology, as described earlier, is a promising step in this new direction, because, in essence, long-term success in chronic-pain management is merely a form of health-behavior training. We hope this new branch of medicine, under the vigorous leadership of John Bonica and other professionals, will soon gain official recognition from the American Medical Association and be granted standards for training and board-certification.

Will efforts such as those outlined above really move us into a pain-free society? Not entirely. The experience of pain, like the phenomenon of death, is an unavoidable part of living. However, the correct application of the laws of behavior and health, when paired with an improved knowledge of pain and its epidemiology, will eventually relieve American society of much of this staggering cost and unacceptable misery. It will increase our productivity and our faith in ourselves, and will justify once again the basic optimism of the American people that they can meet any challenge with practical solutions and lawful process.

PART II

Chronic Pain and the Individual

12

A Personal Commitment to Health May Lead to a Lifestyle Relatively Pain-Free

S. B. CHYATTE

WHEN I WAS A STUDENT in medical school, one of my classmates developed a severe case of viral pneumonia. For days, the young man's life hung in the balance. He was in an oxygen tent, literally struggling for each breath. Finally the crisis was over. On the day he was removed from the oxygen tent, I went to visit him. The first thing the patient did as I entered his room was to light up a cigarette.

Despite his recent battle with death, my classmate had made no personal commitment to health. He, like most of us, returned to his old habits once the immediate danger had passed. We are somehow conditioned to believe that we can do whatever we wish to do with our bodies. If there is no immediate ill effect, we aren't really too worried, but when we do become ill, we want to place ourselves in someone's caring hands. Basically, we seem not to feel a personal responsibility for our own health.

In recent years, more and more attention has been paid by physicians and by the public to the part that diet, exercise, and good living habits play in health. It is increasingly clear that if we are to prevent pain and disease, we must rely heavily on our own efforts.

Obesity is a good example of the need for personal commitment to health. No one knows the miseries of being obese more than a person who is massively overweight. But no one can do anything about it unless the overweight person will take an active role in his own treatment.

This personal commitment to health is critical to those who suffer from chronic pain. Once we get sick, medical care often can restore us to health. But in too many instances, we don't return to our original level of well-being; in these cases, medical care can do little more. We must cope with our remaining problems ourselves. As our poor health grows chronic, we find that more and more responsibility for health care falls on us, the patients—not the doctor.

All the rehabilitation programs mentioned earlier require the patient's willing cooperation. They are successful in helping the patient live a healthier, happier life only to the degree that the individual sufferer makes a personal effort to understand the philosophy and technology involved in his plan of management and fully commits himself to a program of behavioral modification.

There is no point in trying to help a patient function better if he keeps abusing drugs and won't be detoxified. Little success can be expected from a patient who is potentially able to increase his performance levels but refuses to cooperate with his therapist in learning how to improve his muscular skills. There is little chance of relieving postural back pain in a grossly overweight patient who continues to overeat and refuses weight-control therapy.

To understand the part we must play, it is necessary first to be aware of our reactions at various stages of illness. The example of a man who suffers from high blood-pressure will help us review these stages.

At age thirty-five, John C. was found to have high blood-pressure when his physician gave him his yearly physical. He was told to take it easier and relax more, and he was given a low-salt, low-cholesterol diet. He was cautioned to keep his weight down. But John was a busy man. He had a family to feed, a boss who pushed him, and a wife who made the best creamed chicken in town. A ham sandwich with a dill pickle and potato chips was his favorite lunch. And who can find time to exercise while working twelve hours a day?

When he was forty-five, John was twenty pounds overweight and his blood pressure was twenty points higher. His way of life and his eating style were so ingrained that he just couldn't see how he could change. Now he was the boss on his job and worked even harder getting deeply involved in his work.

Still, no one except his physician nagged him. His wife shrugged and said she couldn't change him. Besides, he loved eggs Benedict for breakfast. His teen-aged children lived mostly on their own planet and didn't pay much attention to him. His friends weren't going to tell him what to eat and what to do.

On his forty-seventh birthday, he and his wife celebrated by going out on the town. Returning home at about 2:30 A.M., as they were climbing the stairs to their bedroom, John suddenly grabbed his chest in pain.

Later that night, his doctor informed him he had had an "ischemic attack," a mild heart-attack. As he lay in his hospital bed, John was ready to listen to his doctor's advice. He was scared and realized he must change his ways. His wife was scared, too. Suddenly, cooking creamed chicken wasn't such a wonderful thing; the fur coat she had wanted wasn't so important. Maybe John should take it easier at work, with less emotional involvement.

When he left the hospital, John C. was a new man. He had a diet, a schedule for limiting his work, and was certain he would stick to the new ways. He did—for the first six weeks. There was no more chest pain, and his blood pressure was better. Then he got sick of salt-free food and gradually slipped off his diet. He began to increase his work load, and soon he was back to his old ways.

Two years later he paid the price: a full-fledged myocardial infarction—a no-holds-barred heart attack. It was a full-blown crisis for the family. Everyone was concerned and wanted to do what he or she could. Each chest pain brought worried relatives to his side. John's slightest wish was catered to.

Of course, John couldn't return to work right away after he came home from the hospital. He was too sick even to make out the monthly bills, do any of the housekeeping chores, or anything around the yard.

Gradually, Mrs. C. began to do all the things John had once done. She ran errands in the car, did more of the home-maintenance chores (changing the furnace filter, replacing fuses), and handled the family finances. In sociological terms, she was changing roles; her husband had become the dependent spouse; she was now the dominant one.

Since her children were grown and she needed the income, she got a part-time job. The transition was complete. Mrs. C. was now the family wage-earner.

As time went on, she turned less and less to her husband for advice about her problems. Sick people shouldn't be burdened with making decisions anyway. When she was troubled, she visited her married daughter who lived in their home town, and they talked things over. John was now excluded from his function as head of the family in almost every capacity.

Of course, there was sex. But sick people don't want sex. In fact, it could be dangerous for John. Mrs. C. couldn't tolerate the thought of her husband having another heart attack in the middle of a sexual orgasm. So, by silent mutual agreement, sex was not discussed or engaged in.

John had ceased to be the wage earner, the head of the family, and the sexual partner he had once been. What was his function? His function was to be sick! When you are sick, you don't need to work. Society understands this, and doesn't call you a lazy bum. Society only pities you. When you are sick, no one expects you to trouble yourself with decisions. What kind of car should you buy? Let Mrs. C. pick it out, she's the one who drives it anyway. When you're sick, you can have bad days. So what if you're grumpy; people will understand.

When John was first taken ill, everyone rushed to his aid, but as time wore on, fewer people showed active concern. His children were busy with families of their own. Friends still dropped in, but they were tired of hearing John's complaints. He never seemed to want to do anything anymore. His bowling friends stopped calling. His interests had shrunk to his own problems and himself. He didn't talk about politics or the news, he didn't talk about work; in short, he'd become a pretty boring fellow.

Also, some strange things had happened to his personality. Before his illness, he'd been an easy-going guy; now, at times, he withdrew. Inside himself, he felt guilty. After all, if he'd taken care of himself maybe this wouldn't have happened. Look what he was doing to his wife. He felt like he was a burden to her. What a mess he had made of his life. He was disgusted with himself, yet he seemed unable to change.

Could he return to work? Many sleepless nights he asked himself that question. He was sure he couldn't do the job he had once done. What could he do? Could he work full-time? If he went back to work, his disability check would stop. Could he afford to take that chance? There was also that juicy executive-protection policy that paid him nicely for being unable to work. Would going back to work make him financially better off, or would taxes and other expenses reduce his working income to less than he got now for not working?

When he'd been a busy executive, he hadn't had much time for anyone else. Back then, no one paid much attention to him; he could take care of himself. Now his family looked after him. It was a nice feeling to be cared for. John was receiving what the psychologists call "secondary gain" from his predicament. He was out of the rat-race, being cared for, and had plenty of time to relax! Financially, he didn't have as much as before, but it was coming in without his having to lift a finger.

Also, in the back of his mind, he had a nagging thought. How often, when he'd been well, had he thought, "Boy, if something happened to me, would they be sorry." Well, something had happened, and "they" were sorry. The thought somehow gave him a peculiar sense of satisfaction.

What has happened to John C.? A once perfectly healthy and functional person was taken ill. He should have recovered and resumed a full life. Instead, he fell victim to the "sick role" and played the game of chronic illness. Today, he's a very unhappy person who feels he can't change his life. He's wrong. He *can* change.

Rule One for John C. and for any chronically ill or chronic-pain sufferer: *Keep active and occupied.* While pain in its acute phase is a warning that something is wrong, once you've been thoroughly evaluated and treated, you must often learn to live with the remaining pain. Distraction is one of the best ways of minimizing its perception. When we are chronically ill or in pain, we tend to turn our thoughts toward ourselves, our bodies, our suffering. We intensify our concern and actually increase our perception of our own ills in this manner.

Rule Two: *Direct yourself outward.* Call others who are ill. Make yourself feel concern for them. Consider how your troubles affect those around you. Try to make things easier for them. Get out of your bed and do things, anything, to get away from your inner thoughts.

Illness and pain tend to disrupt our lives, alter our schedules, change our habits. We can't sleep at night so we fall asleep during the day. That makes us less tired at night, and the cycle goes on and on. We don't go to work, so we don't feel the need to get up in the morning. After getting used to sleeping late, we find it difficult to get up early again. Our day begins at 10:00, then 11:00 A.M. Meal schedules are disturbed; bedtime is delayed.

Rule Three: *Maintain a schedule compatible with the rest of the family and the world.* Force yourself to get up as you used to. Shower, dress, and have some purposeful activity planned. Go back to work if possible, if only part-time. Go to the library, the zoo, the local movie theater, but go!

Eat your meals on the family schedule.

We learn to demonstrate our pain to others in many ways. Verbalization or pain complaints are a common method. Pain or sick behavior is another: limping, staying in bed, refusing to lift or bend, taking medicines, etc. Getting others to do things for us when we really could do them ourselves is a third. "Honey, bring me a napkin," you say to your spouse, who is seated as far away from the napkins as you are. "My back hurts when I get up and down too much," you add as your excuse. If pain or sickness is acute, your spouse may be willing, but later, as things get more chronic, such tricks create irritations. Stresses build between the sick person and his family and friends.

Rule Four: *Avoid advertising that you're suffering.* When you've gotten all the medical help you reasonably can expect, you must learn that you're going to have to live with your miseries. Sure, everybody complains occasionally, but it shouldn't be your only source of conversation. You will merely drive everyone away. It doesn't help because it doesn't do anything for your pain.

Many of us have had the experience of trying to cheer up visitors who come to see us when we're sick—people who don't know how to react to our illness. We sometimes have to take the lead and encourage them. It's the same way with chronic illness or pain. It's best to talk about things other than health. We should try to display as little discomfort as possible, because if we don't, we'll soon find ourselves getting fewer and fewer visits. People just feel too uncomfortable listening to others constantly complaining or constantly acting sick. That includes even doctors and nurses.

Pain and illness lead to inactivity, which in turn leads to disuse of muscles, joints, lungs, and heart. These organs become "lazy," and when they're called on to act, they aren't in condition. Weakness, stiffness, and shortness of breath develop. Then, if your mind says "go," your body can't respond.

Rule Five, which needs to be done under the direction of your physician: *Carry on an exercise routine suited to your needs.* This may mean merely walking a certain number of blocks in a set time. It may include flexibility exercises or mild strengthening. No matter what, you must keep up a level of physical activity within your capacity of safety.

The same rules hold true for the chronically ill. You may be physically impaired, but you are only as disabled as you let yourself become. Disability is the effect that impairment has on your ability to do things. If you're still able to work, you are not disabled even if both arms have been cut off and you are blind.

Pain is a part of life. It can be a constructive experience if we meet the challenge and commit ourselves to a healthy lifestyle, despite the hurt we feel. But many of us are using pain in a destructive manner, not only harmful to ourselves but to our whole society. When pain is used to avoid responsibilities, shun work, gain attention, and excuse failure, it destroys the individual who has the pain, disrupts families, and tears at the fabric of society.

In the Pain Control Center at Emory University, patient after patient says, "I want to go back to work." After evaluation and treatment, the patient is told, "You can return to work." The patient then gets furious. "What do you mean, I can go back to work? I'm sick!"

Actually these patients aren't faking; they're fooling themselves. When a patient says he wants to go back to work, he really is saying, "I want to be like I was before I got sick." If he truly wants to go back to work, he wants to return to his old job or to a better job. Not a new or modified one. He doesn't just want to work, he has a specific set of work conditions in mind. But it may not be possible to meet these conditions. When we get sick or injured, we must learn a new image of ourselves, for we have changed. The professional football player with the torn knee must seek another way to earn his livelihood. The factory worker with back pain may have to learn a new trade.

We are increasingly aware of the importance of ecology in sustaining a healthy environment. The ecology of man is equally important. We can't afford to waste the precious natural resources of our land, and neither can we afford to waste individuals. When a person ceases to function, to be productive, we all lose something. We must recycle our disabled workers. If each of us grows dependent on someone else, who will be left to support us all?

EDITOR'S NOTE: *The physician who contributed this chapter, Dr. Chyatte, adds the following personal comment: "You may think I'm just another doctor talking—a healthy person who at worst has an occasional backache. Let me set you straight: I've been there! I'm partially paralyzed in my arms and legs, and a diabetic who depends on an artificial kidney for life. Pain and physical impairment are daily events to me. My own rules have worked for me. It hasn't been easy but it's been worth it. You have to really want to fight your disability. You have to have a personal commitment to your own health, if you want to live relatively happy, in a state of peace of mind and productivity.*

13

The Anatomy of Pain

S. F. BRENA

THIS SECTION of the book is focused on chronic pain in relation to the individual sufferer. It is our belief that the victim of chronic pain, armed with the proper knowledge and attitude, can help greatly in alleviating his own suffering.

First, we'll present some basic information on the workings of the nervous and muscle systems, and how each system deciphers and communicates both acute and chronic pain.

Then we'll explore some relatively new but promising techniques for dealing with chronic pain without resorting to excessive drug use or heroic surgical intervention.

Finally, we will explore the most common specific painful experiences that afflict modern man, and we'll report on the current state of the art in coping with these experiences, from the point of view of both the sufferer and the medical profession.

Space technology, with all its sophisticated machinery, is like a child's toy when compared with the millions of circuits, switchboards, circuit-breakers, feedback loops, and command stations that form man's central nervous system, all neatly and compactly organized within the tiny space of our skull and spinal column.

Today's scientist is granted only a tiny glimpse of the marvelous flow of energy along these nerve circuits when he implants electrodes into the nervous system, to monitor and record on an oscilloscope the endless sequences of light waves that are the intimate expression of what we really are: waves of energy-light. We are reminded of the Book of Genesis: "And God said, let there be light, and there was light."

A cornerstone of the nervous system is the nerve cell, or neuron, which has one or more appendages, called nerve fibers. There are various groups of nerve fibers: some with relatively large diameters (A-fibers), others with smaller diameters (C-fibers); some covered by a protective sheath, others unprotected. Nerve fibers can be thought of as electrical cables that transmit information in two directions: from the periphery of the body to the spinal cord and brain through afferent, or inflowing, impulses; and from the brain to appropriate organs, such as muscles and glands, through outflowing, or efferent, impulses. The impulses traveling along these nerve fibers can actually be seen and recorded as light waves. The large fibers transmit impulses at a relatively high speed, between 15 and 120 meters per second; the small fibers conduct at much lower speeds, between 0.5 and 1.0 meter per second.

Another cornerstone of the nervous system is the "synapse," which can be thought of as a relay organ, a place of contact between two nerve cells, where an impulse is electrochemically transmitted from one cell to another. The synapse can also be viewed as an extremely tiny switchboard or circuit-breaker that can open or close nerve circuits. Both the neuron and the synapse are being studied intensively to learn more about their respective roles in "patterning" impulse sequences that can be perceived by the brain as particular sensory experiences.

Both these structures seem able, by repetitive activity within particular areas of the central nervous system, to store the memory of impulse patterns along nerve circuits. Sir John Eccles, the neurophysiologist and Nobel Prize winner, has called these programmed nerve-cell circuits "engrams." He has proposed the engram concept to explain our memory.

In contrast to the "pattern" theory of nerve activity and its view that the nervous system is an electronic-type machine that is programmed like a computer, other theories look at the nervous system as an electrically wired apparatus with specific, fixed circuits designed to carry the same kind of information in a static, prearranged fashion, rather than in a dynamic, ever-changing pattern.

The German physiologist Johannes Müller was the first to propose a "theory of specific nerve energy," in 1826. According to him, stimulation of a given sense organ gives rise to its own particular sensation and no other. Pain was viewed in terms of Müller's ideas of nerve specificity from the mid-nineteenth century until a few years ago. It was regarded as a specific sensation caused by particular stimuli which activate specialized sense organs.

In the past decade, however, improved studies have redefined and reclassified our various senses into new groupings based on their initial physical-energy sources.

Specialized structures called receptors have been identified in the skin and in other sensitive body tissues; these receptors are capable of converting certain types of energy into nerve impulses. Our sense of vision, for example, is generated by light receptors in the retina that convert heat and electromagnetic energy into nerve impulses.

Some receptors, widely distributed on the surface of the body as well as in deeper body structures and in the viscera, do not respond to nonharmful stimulation, but only to mechanical and heat stimuli of such intensity as to cause tissue damage. These receptors are called nociceptors and are capable of converting into nerve impulses changes that threaten the integrity of body organs. Nociceptors can be viewed as the first link in a long chain of neurological events that eventually lead to the pain experience and response.

Nerve impulses that carry information about tissue damage are called nociceptive impulses. It must be emphasized that these impulses are not the real thing—the pain experience as we all know it. They are merely an electrochemical activity along certain peripheral nerve-pathways. Only when nociceptive impulses reach the integrative central-brain area are they perceived as pain. Nature has probably designed nociceptive impulses to be perceived as highly unpleasant, so that they will trigger quick protective action to stop further body damage. Quite rightly, Sir Charles Sherrington has called the perception of pain "a psychological adjunct of an imperative, protective reflex," the result of a conflict between the stimulus and the individual.

A distortion of this protective mechanism, which shows that the pain experience is not merely a sensation but an integrated central perception, is seen in people who actually regard nociceptive impulses as pleasant. Such people often submit gladly to body-damaging insults such as being whipped and chained; some of these maladjusted individuals stick needles into their own flesh and claim to feel physical and sexual pleasure. This well-known phenomenon is called masochism; its counterpart, in people who enjoy inflicting pain on others, is sadism.

In common language, nociceptive impulses may also be referred to as "painful" or "pain-producing" impulses. Such terms will be used throughout this book, but the reader should understand that they are not precisely accurate in a scientific sense.

The pain-producing impulses mentioned above travel toward the brain along at least two different nerve-fiber networks. One set of impulses moves rapidly to the cerebral cortex—two hemispheres located at the outermost layers of the brain—via the fast-conducting, large-fiber pathway, with few synaptic relays along the way. It is this faster system that scientists consider to be a step higher on the evolutionary ladder of life.

A second set of painful impulses is transmitted centrally along the small-fiber network. This network has many complex synaptic relays all along the spinal cord and in the inner brain areas known as the reticular formation, the thalamus, and the hypothalamus. This network has fewer fibers reaching directly to the higher brain centers.

Recent studies in neuroanatomy indicate that there are other fiber networks capable of picking up pain-producing impulses in particular distress situations. These studies are not yet complete, however, and their significance is not clear.

A good way to think of the two systems mentioned above is as follows: If you accidentally put your hand on a steaming pot of coffee, you will first notice a quick, burning sensation, localized in your burned hand. This tells you immediately that you've been injured and must take action to avoid further damage. A few seconds later, you will feel another unpleasant sensation, much less localized, which spreads from your injured hand up toward your arm, setting the whole arm "on fire." This second sensation is less likely to trigger quick action, but it does prompt you to voice your pain with a curse, moan, groan, or whatever emotional expression you've learned to use when hurt.

The first sensation rapidly reached your cerebral hemispheres via the large-fiber, few-relays system: It has the specific function of warning you to take protective action. The second feeling was carried along the small-fiber, multirelay network, which has a tendency—because of its many relays—to spread impulses and trigger emotions. The two sets of nerve networks carrying painful information seem related to each other in a kind of check-and-balance system that is described scientifically by the "gate-control" theory.

According to this now-famous theory, first proposed by Ronald Melzack and Patrick Wall in 1965, the large-fiber system has the function of screening small-fiber input in a specific area of the spinal cord known as the spinal gate. Stimulation of the large fibers will cause an overload of large-fiber traffic and result in fewer small-fiber impulses getting through the gate. An example of the way this works is the following: After you have burned your hand on a hot coffee-pot, you are likely to feel some relief if you vigorously rub your wrist and squeeze your forearm. What are you doing? You are overloading large-fiber input with tactile or "touch" impulses that are also carried by the large nerve-fibers. This phenomenon is the basis for an effective method of pain relief called transcutaneous electrical nerve stimulation (TENS), which will be discussed in Chapter Eighteen.

There is evidence that the transmission of painful impulses is also under the control of various waves of nerve impulses traveling from the higher brain areas down toward the so-called spinal gate. These descending control systems exercise a great deal of screening at the spinal-cord level, opening or closing the gate according to the amount of activity at the gate.*

One particular brain structure, the limbic system, seems deeply involved in the painful experience. Anatomically, various brain centers, including the thalamus and hypothalamus, are grouped under this name; they are known to be "receiving stations" for painful impulses. The limbic system forms a ring around the upper brain-stem, at the inner core of the central nervous system. It is an older brain structure, common to all mammals, and is also called the visceral brain. It controls a large number of vital visceral functions and provides for the expression of emotions through the activation of the sympathetic nervous system. (The sympathetic and parasympathetic nervous systems will be discussed in the next chapter).

The limbic system is linked to those areas of the brain called the neocortex. A much younger brain structure in terms of evolution, the neocortex has developed to a large size only in man: It can properly be viewed as the highest command station in humans. The entire thinking and

* EDITOR'S NOTE: *The "Spinal Gate Theory" is presently under intense research, scrutiny and criticism. The "check and balance" system of fiber networks may be even more complex than the theory itself postulates. However, the "Gate Theory" has served a tremendously useful purpose in challenging Müller's idea of energy of specific nerves, and has focused our attention more precisely as to the role of the spinal cord and of the central nervous system, where the individual painful perception originates.*

performance behaviors of an individual are related to the proper functioning of the neocortex.

We know that the neocortex serves to integrate various nerve activities, particularly within the limbic and autonomic systems. When man is in command of his visceral and emotional functions through proper neocortical monitoring—a learned, intelligent process—the resulting behaviors are well-integrated and adapted to achieve any goal.

But when man lowers his command post to the visceral brain because of failure to use his neocortical abilities, his daily life is controlled by his feelings and is no longer balanced by intelligent thinking. His sympathetic nervous activities are upset, muscle tension increases, and various maladjusted behaviors follow. In the face of challenge, defense mechanisms fail and multiple miseries are born. Chronic pain and chronic sickness are among them.

14

Pain and Vital Functions

W. D. HAMMONDS

WE TELL THOSE AROUND US that we hurt by what we say and do. But, as we have seen, these signals of pain can be grossly inaccurate, because emotional factors often cloud the issue. Aside from injury or illness, there are other, less socially acceptable reasons for skipping school or work or for taking narcotic pain relievers.

An entirely different set of signals communicates the expression of pain from within and may be detected by the careful observer. These signals are generated by many organ systems, but all are linked together by the autonomic nervous system, which supports all vital functions of the body. There are two major divisions of the autonomic system: the sympathetic and the parasympathetic.

Anatomically, the sympathetic system is composed of a

vast network of fine nerve-fibers that are connected with the spinal cord through relays called sympathetic ganglia, located all along the vertebral column. From these spinal ganglia, sympathetic fibers go out to supply almost every bodily organ.

The parasympathetic section of the autonomic system is an older, more primitive system in terms of human evolution, with fewer fiber networks and relays. Its main component is the vitally important vagus nerve, which originates in a brain area called the brain stem, located toward the rear and base of the skull, where other important stations for the control of vital functions are located. From the brain stem, the vagus nerve goes out to supply fibers to the heart, lungs, stomach, bowels, and other organs.

The sympathetic system triggers invigorating mechanisms that make us ready for "fight or flight." Sympathetic action, for instance, may speed up the heart rate, whereas the parasympathetic system slows it down. In another example, bowel movements are impaired by sympathetic overactivity, but they are smoothed by the action of the vagus nerve. Obviously, we need increased heart performance while fighting or running away, but we do not need to take in food at the same time. The two sections of the autonomic nervous system, acting in opposite directions, help to maintain the body's homeostasis—that state of affairs in which the internal biochemical reactions of the healthy body are kept in balance. This balance is necessary to regulate the composition of body fluids, to maintain a constant temperature, and to control secretions of hormones from many glands so that life can go on.

The function of the autonomic nervous system is evaluated indirectly by checking the so-called vital signs. Pulse, temperature, respiration, and blood pressure are the classic vital signs, but information about activity in the autonomic nervous system can also be obtained from perspiration, skin color, and the psycho-galvanic reflex (an electronic method of measuring skin resistance, which rises when the individual is in a relaxed state and goes down measurably with anxiety).

When a painful injury occurs, the heart rate increases, providing greater force to make the blood circulate faster. There is an almost simultaneous deepening of respirations, delivering more oxygen to the lungs, where it can be picked up by the already-augmented circulation. There is a reflex relaxation of the smooth muscles surrounding the tiny air passages in the lungs, making possible the movement of even greater volumes of air with each breath. All of these changes following the sudden onset of pain prepare the heart and respiratory system to fight or run in those situations in which a threat, real or imagined, is perceived.

Other changes prepare the body for massive physical exertion. There is a shift of blood flow from the internal organs and skin to the skeletal muscles, heart, and brain. This movement of blood away from the skin accounts for the pallor so commonly observed in acute pain. The diversion of blood from internal organs brings a profound slowing of digestion. There are changes in the circulating blood that can be detected only by laboratory analysis. More red blood-cells are expelled from storage and placed in the circulating blood. Since red blood-cells function primarily to carry oxygen, the body is made increasingly more capable of meeting the demands of great physical stress.

The blood-sugar level also rises immediately. The reason for this is that sugar is the basic fuel of the body's muscle system. Even the eye is affected by pain. Any man who has nicked himself with a razor and then looked at himself in the shaving mirror can attest that there is a sudden dilation of the eye. This helps change the eye's focus from a near to a far object and might have value in looking into the distance—to visualize an escape route from the origin of the pain.

Injury is not always followed by activation of the sympathetic system. In humans, an overwhelmingly painful experience may activate the parasympathetic system instead, with slowing of the pulse, decrease in blood pressure, and occasional fainting. Such parasympathetic responses to injury and distress are seen mostly in association with injuries to the intestines or other internal organs, and may be viewed as a protective reaction that influences the injured person to be inactive rather than struggle.

Pain is not alone in producing this variety of bodily changes: Fear and anxiety produce similar changes. In fact, it is often impossible to separate changes caused by fear and anxiety from changes caused by pain.

Looked at in terms of evolution, fear and rage have generated useful survival reflexes in the development of the human race. Fear is associated with an overpowering desire to escape the offending object or person. The wild animal that attacked primitive man was thereafter avoided because of fear. Meanwhile, an unprovoked attack by an enemy evoked rage. A more effective defense could thus be mounted because of strength derived from rage. This is why, today, accidents and injuries are always followed by a great outpouring of strong emotions in victims which themselves may cause both sympathetic and parasympathetic responses. Arousal of the autonomic nervous system and changes in vital functions after a painful experience have beneficial effects in the sense that they prepare the body to meet the challenge of whatever has triggered the painful episode.

However, when the autonomic arousal is excessive and uncontrolled, the results are harmful. A good example of this is the way such arousal can inhibit the smooth progression of labor in a pain-prone pregnant woman. The expulsive contractions of the uterus can be made more effective by giving the woman enough medication to abate the pain; even more effective is the administration of a properly applied regional anesthetic. Natural childbirth techniques also call for the husband's presence to reassure and help the expectant mother control her body's responses to the pain experience. Other examples of harmful effects from the uncontrolled arousal of the sympathetic system are high blood-pressure and constipation, which are often associated with states of anxiety and pain.

In the evolutionary development of the human race, man faced many physical dangers. Those people who gained additional strength to fight enemies or to kill animals for food through autonomic nervous-system activation were the ones who survived. And those who survived passed their genes on to succeeding offspring. After countless generations, the surviving race is well-endowed with nervous-system mechanisms that supply additional margins of strength when needed.

But in our modern society, when so often the reactions of pain, fear, and rage cannot be acted out by "fight or flight," such emotions may express themselves physically as ulcers or high blood-pressure. It is tempting to speculate that techniques such as meditation and biofeedback training will play an important role in the prevention and treatment of such problems by helping the sufferer to control and pacify his own autonomic nervous system.

15

Pain and Muscles

S. F. BRENA

MUSCLES ARE BODY-STRUCTURES capable of tightening and relaxing; they are responsible for countless things that people do, including the skillful play of an artist's hands on a piano keyboard, the rasping voice of a drill sergeant, the superb performance of an Olympic athlete, the beating of a heart, the expulsion of a fetus from a uterus, the blinking of an eye, and the widening and narrowing of arteries and veins.

Some muscles (the skeletal or striated type) are controlled by will power; others (smooth muscles) have an inherent rhythmic contraction—the heart muscle, for example. But even the smooth muscles can be brought under conscious control to a degree by techniques such as meditation and biofeedback training.

Without muscular function, we would not be able to communicate or survive. In most mammals and men, skeletal muscles make up half the body weight and use most of the energy created by the body. Actually, our pattern of energy metabolism is determined almost entirely by our skeletal muscles.

Just as the neuron is a basic feature of the nervous system, the muscle cell with its "motor-end plate," where the nerve-fiber joins the muscle cell, is a cornerstone of the muscular system. In the striated (skeletal) muscles, cells are elongated and fuse-shaped along the line of contraction: their contractile properties are derived from special proteins that are the main part of the cell.

Several muscle cells may be "fired" by one neuron or nerve cell; the group of muscle cells under control of a single neuron is called a "motor unit." A whole muscle contains a number of motor units along with sensory nerve-fibers attached to nerve receptors within the substance of the muscle, and blood vessels that supply oxygen to the muscle and remove the waste of metabolic combustion.

The fibers of the smooth, visceral muscles are smaller than those of striated muscles. These fibers are found in the walls of various hollow organs—stomach, bowels, blood vessels, etc. Usually, visceral fibers are arranged in two sets, an inner core of fibers circularly arranged and an outer shell that is oriented lengthwise.

Just as the activity of nerves can be recorded by an electrical device, so will an electrode placed on or inserted into a muscle detect the electrical activity of adjacent motor units. We see this as a light-wave pattern in the electromyograph (EMG).

Muscles contract in two different ways. If the attachments (tendons) of the muscle are fixed, the contractile activity shapes into tension without actual movement; this contraction is called isometric. On the other hand, if one or both tendons can move, the muscle shortens without tension and generates a movement; this second type of contraction is called isotonic. In a healthy, well-trained muscle, isometric and isotonic contractions are always balanced so as to obtain maximum work with a minimum expenditure of energy. For instance, in lifting a heavy object, you will first apply isometric tension to the muscles of your arm to get the object off the floor; you will then use mostly isotonic contractions to further lift the object and perform your work.

Muscle groups that work together to generate a movement are called synergistic; those that fix the body's position as a whole to facilitate group muscular movements are called postural. Even in the simplest movement, an intricate balance between isometric and isotonic contractions and between synergistic and postural muscles is set in motion. This is accomplished by rapid-firing, reflex nerve-circuits, running to and from the spinal cord and brain, which direct the whole operation in that fraction of a second you require, for example, to clench your fist.

Devices to eliminate friction are provided wherever a muscle or tendon rubs against another anatomical structure. Each of these devices is called a bursa; it is simply a collapsed bag with thin, moist, slippery walls. When a tendon runs between other structures in tunnel-like fashion, as in the hands and feet, the bursa may surround the tendon to form a synovial sheath; this helps avoid friction on all sides. Both the bursae and synovial sheaths can get inflamed and cause a great deal of painful stimulation.

In a healthy, relaxed muscle, there is no detectable electrical activity on the EMG. However, few of us are capable of putting our muscles into a total resting position at will. Most of our muscles are never completely at rest; more often than not, a muscle "tone" is detectable by electrical monitoring even when we are pretending to relax. Actually, this so-called muscle tone is not a function of the muscle itself, but a state of irritability in the nervous system controlling the skeletal muscles. Rightly, we can think of the muscle tone as a tremendous waste of energy, which may partially explain why people who do not know how to relax often feel tired and worn out. Muscle fibers that have lost their nerve supply, however, continue to show multiple contractions, detectable by EMG recording.

When muscles are fatigued, they fail to relax; the subjective equivalent of a stretched muscle is a "muscle spasm." Muscular fatigue is due to an accumulation of acid lactates within the muscle substance. These lactates, which are basically combustion waste, increase as the oxygen supply to the muscle decreases under sustained tension; this is roughly equivalent to the way smoke increases in a fire with poor draught. Poor "draught" conditions in our body tissues are called hypoxia (low oxygen). A fatigued or hypoxic muscle is a painful muscle; lactates are known to be irritants capable of activating pain receptors in the muscle itself and of setting off volleys of painful impulses to the spinal cord and brain.

If this state of irritability and acute pain is not promptly corrected by efficient muscular relaxation, a dangerous circular movement is triggered. Both the brain and spinal cord, when bombarded by painful impulses, respond with waves of motor impulses that result in more sustained muscle tension. This in turn produces more lactates, because of improper combustion. Soon the sympathetic nervous system gets involved, setting off nerve impulses to the blood vessels in the affected area. Too much activity of the sympathetic system causes a constriction of the small arteries to all the muscles within a particular anatomical region, further decreasing the oxygen supply. Lactates increase as more groups of hypoxic muscles are recruited. The result is overloaded pain-producing traffic on nerve pathways, which may finally break down or overcome the modulating action of the "spinal gate" and establish a chronic-pain state.

Finally, muscles under deranged metabolic conditions, lacking proper function, lose their ability to contract and relax. They become swollen (edematous) and stiff. Various abnormal materials accumulate among the muscle cells, including blood platelets and the mucopolysaccharides, such as heparin. These materials freeze the muscle in a clinical disorder called fibrositis. In the first chapter, we mentioned disuse as one of the Five D's—the five most common consequences of chronic pain. Muscle fibrositis is the most frequently seen of the various disuse lesions; it is a very troublesome problem when efforts are made to rehabilitate people with chronic pain to live a more relaxed and functional life.

The circular movement just described, or "vicious circle of pain" as W. K. Livingston called it a quarter of a century ago, can begin at any point in the circle. At the muscular level, injury, disease, or habitually poor posture can trigger it. Many back pains have their origin in chronic fibrositis of the back muscles. This is often caused by chronic strain of the spine's postural muscles because of overweight with bulging abdomen, or faulty body postures from inadequate exercise and immobility.

At the level of the vertebral column, injury of the vertebral joints, osteoarthritis, and other vertebral defects can trigger the "vicious circle" via overactive reflex nerve-circuits. The whiplash injury, frequently associated with traffic accidents, particularly rear-end-type collisions, often becomes permanently painful because of sprain of the vertebral joints and reactive, diffuse fibrositis. Visceral diseases such as myocardial infarction (heart attack), endocrine disturbances such as diabetes, and allergic reactions can trigger the fibrositis-disuse syndrome.

At the psychological level, emotional stress, secondary gain, and various other personality maladjustments, spurred on by chronic anxiety, depression, and behavioral conditioning, can cause increased nervous muscle tone and set the stage for a circular movement of chronic muscular pain. This may be started by seemingly minor factors such as a common cold or weather changes from warm-and-dry to cold-and-wet.

Emotional and personality factors are important in a variety of visceral disorders—they act by increasing tone in the smooth muscles lining the walls of hollow organs. The so-called irritable or spastic colon is a common psychosomatic illness in which emotional forces are converted into severe malfunction of the colon, with runaway constipation and abdominal discomfort. Other well-known psychosomatic ailments are certain forms of gastritis, some changes in heart function, menstrual troubles, and high blood-pressure in the absence of detectable organic causes.

Spinal reflexes also sometimes link the striated and smooth muscles so that abnormal function in one set of muscles may spill over to the other set via multiple synaptic nerve-relays in the spinal cord. If you have suffered an episode of acute appendicitis, you will remember an exquisite tenderness and rigidity in the voluntary muscles of the lower right quadrant of your abdomen. This is a good example of a spinal reflex action in which your inflamed intestinal appendix triggered waves of pain-producing nerve impulses to the spinal cord. These impulses "spilled over" the spinal gate at various levels, and set in motion painful impulses to the muscles and blood vessels in the lower abdominal wall, which lies over the appendix site.

There is evidence that breathing rates, sympathetic nerve activity, and muscle tension are all linked together, probably in the reticular formation. This formation, a crossroads of nerve pathways at the inner core of the brain, binds together the totality of our body functions. Changes in breathing rates trigger volleys of impulses over sympathetic nerves, resulting in changes of blood flow to various muscle groups. The nervous irritability generated by rapid breathing may also directly upset muscle tone. On the other hand, slow-breathing rhythms are known to be conducive to muscular relaxation, possibly through a decrease of nerve impulses to the muscles and blood vessels.

Our present knowledge of anatomy and physiology confirms the old Greek concept of human wholeness in both mind and body. Each organ and function is linked to all others in intimate, delicate balance. Any disease process affecting one organ or body system is likely to spill over and affect the whole mind-body unit. The control or elimination of any given disease process will not necessarily restore complete health and normal function, unless the individual in his or her wholeness is helped toward total mind-body recovery.

16

Behavior Modification to Control Chronic Pain

I. P. UNIKEL

MRS. MARY A., a forty-five-year-old homemaker, complained of low-back pain, visited physicians often, and was a heavy user of pills. She had had two back operations with little relief. Because of her frequent complaints, her physician contemplated another operation but decided to refer her to a pain-control center first.

At the center, she was put on a "contingency management" program that allowed her only limited use of drugs for pain. Her activities were monitored carefully for a week, and it was found she spent much of her time in bed or watching television. She was active less than two hours a day and did not complete her household chores and other work.

She was asked to increase her activities at least thirty minutes each week above her previous week's level during a six-week program, with continuous monitoring of her performance. If she did as instructed (and only when she did) she would be given medical treatment for pain relief—in this case a nerve block.

By the end of a six-week period of contingency management, Mrs. A. had become active for ten to twelve hours each day; this included exercise, household chores such as preparation of meals, and other activities such as shopping and bowling. She returned for follow-up visits at one-month and six-month intervals after discharge from the pain clinic. It was found that she was essentially still as active as when discharged from the program. Also, she had not consulted with doctors about her chronic pain during this time.

Not all patients show gains of such impressive magnitude as Mrs. A. However, about 65 percent of chronic sufferers who receive contingency management do show significant improvement. These cases include helpless patients who were previously crippled by chronic pain, with past histories involving unsuccessful surgeries for pain and multiple-drug misuse. After treatment they were able to go back to normal personal maintenance and household chores, social and recreational activities, and even to paid employment. It has been found that these programs, if carried through to a successful conclusion, result in patients feeling less physical pain and more physically fit. They increase well-being, self-esteem, and personal happiness.

The principles of operant conditioning are involved here. The idea is to make a goal desired by the patient contingent on activities that will lead to improved health and adjustment. Meanwhile, undesirable behavior is eliminated: Drug abuse and excessive verbalization of pain, for example, are not rewarded.

The usual practice in medical settings in the past has been to allow patients to take drugs as needed. This is often done by giving the patient a bottle of pills to be taken when pain is felt, and drugs are frequently prescribed when the patient convinces the doctor that there is pain. In these instances, the medication is contingent on pain behavior and may serve to reward and perpetuate it. Such practices often lead to overreliance on pills, with consequent addiction.

Wilbert Fordyce has pointed out that similar problems occur when beneficial activities and exercise are prescribed for patients, but at the same time, the patients are told to rest when they've done all they can tolerate, or told to decide when to return to work. In such settings, patients are left on their own to determine when to quit. In these conditions, rest becomes contingent on hurting. The sooner there is pain, the quicker the patient can let up. Moreover, the pain is followed by a pleasant state of rest that tends to serve as a reward for the pain behavior. In fact, stopping to rest is reinforced because it eases the pain.

Contingency-management programs for drugs and activities are based on the same principles in reverse. Drugs are prescribed on a basis that does not involve a reward or otherwise encourage the occurrence of pain behavior. One way to accomplish this is by prescribing the medication at specified time intervals, regardless of when pain occurs, so that the drug is independent of pain behavior. Likewise, activities are prescribed in specific amounts that are based on careful, reliable observations of the patient's capabilities at a given time. Patients are trained to adjust their activity levels according to instructions received from the therapist, not according to their own feelings.

In programs of behavior modification such as these, rewards are programmed systematically to follow behavioral changes that contribute to the patient's health. Elimination of sick behavior is matched by conditioning with more adaptive and socially desirable behaviors. Improvement in specific behaviors usually results in general improvement in the patient's lifestyle: He learns that he can control himself and his environment again. The major focus in the most successful programs for chronic pain has been to encourage the chronic patient, by use of these techniques, to get out of bed and lead as active a life as possible.

In a typical, comprehensive, contingency-management treatment program, patients are given specific daily assignments to perform such as exercise, walking, sports, or household chores. Each patient is given tasks within the limits of his capabilities, with precedence going to activities he enjoys or would like to do. It is understood that the activities must be carried out for a prescribed amount of time before they are given medical treatment for pain relief. Therefore the giving of a pain-relief procedure is contingent on the performance of the necessary activities. As the treatment continues, the patient is required to become progressively more active until a suitable level of activity is reached.

A related problem is anxiety and its associated physical tension, which account for a great deal of aggravation of pain problems. Aside from their direct physiological effects and the increased suffering they cause, anxiety and tension may lead to conditioned pain behavior far in excess of the physical disease itself. Drugs that relieve anxiety, such as Valium, usually do provide some relief of painful feelings as well: When pain is acute and anxiety high, the tranquilizing drugs are useful in making the patient comfortable. They help him cope with his acute problem more efficiently.

However, in cases of chronic anxiety, the prolonged use of tranquilizers can also produce opposite effects. As seen earlier, these drugs, when not used properly, induce drowsiness, uncoordinated movements, and impaired judgment. The result is a decrease in coping mechanisms and an increase in feelings of insecurity, helplessness, and anxiety. Thus, while untreated anxiety can be a major factor in development of chronic-pain states, attempts to treat chronic anxiety with tranquilizers will often only compound the pain problem.

Patients can learn how to relax without drugs, and thus be helped with both acute and chronic pain problems. Specific methods of relaxation training, such as the Jacobson exercises and biofeedback, are discussed in a later chapter. Such methods are most successful when they are part of an overall contingency-management program. In such a program, participation by the patient in the practice of how to relax and reduce tension can be assured, because desired rewards and successful completion of the program are made contingent on performance of these activities as well as others.

The patient is involved in a comprehensive treatment effort that enables him to cope better with life's problems. He learns to avoid the disruptive effects of anxiety by relaxing when it occurs. The patient who is successful in relaxation procedures gains another behavioral technique to use in times of anxiety and distress; he does not have to take tranquilizing drugs and sleeping pills.

17

Relaxation Techniques to Control Pain

S. L. CHAPMAN AND
C. N. SHEALY

MUCH RELIEF IN CHRONIC PAIN can be achieved simply by learning how to relax tense muscles. This can be accomplished by various steps. First, good oxygen supply to poorly functioning, disused muscles must be reestablished by improving blood flow in painful areas. Safe techniques are now available to carry greater amounts of oxygen to the tissues and wash out lactates and other irritant materials. For example, sympathetic-nerve blocks and electrical nerve stimulation are good methods to increase regional blood flow and provide temporary relief from chronic pain.

A second step in the functional reeducation of disused muscles is physical and occupational therapy under the supervision of a therapist. Exercises learned with professional supervision, such as the Williams exercises for low-back pain, can be routinely performed at home.

A third and very important step in functional reeducation consists of training the patient to reestablish a normal—or as close to normal as possible—pattern of desired activities. For instance, it is imperative that patients with muscle and nerve disorders such as spinal-cord injuries learn muscle skills that will make them independent in daily hygiene tasks. Other patients are often gratified to learn how to overcome muscular stiffness from osteoarthritis, and to be reeducated to carry on social, recreational, and sexual activities. Getting back to normal activities helps relieve depression and keeps patients from being overwhelmed by their chronic pain.

A fourth step consists of actually teaching the individual how to relax. You have probably heard friends tell you, "Relax!" Without proper training, however, you can no more relax than you can fly without taking flying lessons. Many individuals do not even know when their muscles are not relaxed. It seems the brain often turns off its perception of tension when stress is constant. However, stress and its accompanying muscle tension continue to cause or worsen psychosomatic disorders and aggravate emotional distress. Thus, one of the first steps necessary in teaching relaxation is to make the patient aware of tension and its harmful effects. Once he is aware of the problem, the individual needs to learn that he has the power to control it. He can be taught to abandon his self-pity and learned helplessness for a condition of hope and self-reliance. Finally, he needs to be able to perceive when he is beginning to get tense and to release his tension immediately through relaxation techniques.

All these techniques are useful in preventing tension build-up, but they are less effective when begun after the patient has reached such a highly anxious state that he can't concentrate or divert himself from bodily discomfort. Tense muscles don't relax easily; even sleep is usually not the answer. Many people with stressful lives keep their muscles tight all night long, and dreaming can further increase the tension. In difficult situations, whether real or imagined, these patients are caught in a vicious cycle of increased pain and tension.

How can a person gain self-control over bodily functions? We will discuss six techniques which have proved useful in large numbers of patients: counseling, meditation, biofeedback training, progressive relaxation, autogenic training, and mental training exercises.

Counseling. Many individuals are in need of counseling about harmful life patterns, attitudes, and thoughts. These patients spend much of their time worrying about what might happen to themselves or to others. They imagine situations that might cause them difficulty, even though such situations are not likely to happen and would probably be manageable if they did occur.

Treatment for such individuals may need to focus on changing the basic insecurity or low self-esteem that underlies these concerns, as well as on teaching the patient to think more positively and to "take life as it comes." If these sources of tension are not dealt with, the direct modification of bodily processes through relaxation or biofeedback techniques may prove unsuccessful. Professional counseling can be provided by primary physicians, clinical psychologists, and psychiatrists, or by other qualified health professionals.

Meditation. Bodily functions that are associated with tension and anxiety are largely governed by the autonomic nervous system. Traditionally, the autonomic system has been described as working outside of self-awareness; it was once considered independent of mind and will, as the name "autonomic" implies. Recent research, however, suggests that autonomic functions are not beyond conscious control. Adherents of Zen Buddhism and Yoga have long claimed that by meditation—and by commitment to a lifestyle conducive to proper meditation—they can enter an altered state of consciousness in which their heart rate and breathing are governed by the mind. One currently popular technique of meditation is called transcendental meditation (TM); it involves spending a period of time each day in a meditative state while mentally focusing on a word or phrase known as a mantra, which is personal to the individual.

One of the first scientific investigations of the meditative process came in 1935, when Thérèse Brosse, a French cardiologist, tested meditating yogis with electrocardiographic equipment. She concluded that one of her subjects could actually stop his heart while meditating. Later investigators cast doubt on this finding, but they did measure the slowing down of the heart and breathing rates in yogis. Recent studies have shown that subjects really do slow their metabolism, raise skin temperature, increase blood flow, and slow their breathing during meditation. These abilities seem to reflect a conscious control over the autonomic nervous system.

Biofeedback Training. Biofeedback means exactly what the name implies—it provides information, or "feedback," about biological processes. It uses technology to train people to control body functions. In biofeedback training, some device that measures a body function such as muscle tension, heart rate, or skin temperature, is placed on the body of the individual being treated. The patient is thus provided information, perhaps by means of a light, a sound, or a digital display, about how much tension he has, how fast his heart is beating, or how warm his skin temperature is. He is then given instructions on how to modify the body process, and his performance is measured with the biofeedback device.

Gradually, the patient learns what he has to do to control the body process in question, and with practice at home, he learns to prevent harmful processes from occurring. For example, the tension-headache patient can learn to tell when the muscles that cause his headache are getting tense and learn what he needs to do to reduce the tension. Muscle spasms and other muscular dysfunctions that result in chronic pain often can similarly be brought under control of the patient.

With some of the newest technology, almost every physiological process can be monitored, amplified, and fed back to conscious awareness, permitting the patient to learn to bring his functions to normal levels. Pulse rate; blood pressure; skin temperature (an expression of blood circulation); electrocardiogram (EKG); electromyograph (EMG); electroencephalogram (EEG), or brain-wave frequency; pressure changes in the eyes; and many other bodily functions have been brought into healthier ranges by use of biofeedback braining.

Progressive Relaxation. It is generally recognized that many symptoms and illnesses are either directly or indirectly a result of emotional stress. As stated by F. J. Ingelfinger, 80 percent of illnesses are either self-limited or not treatable by modern medicine and surgery. Despite such knowledge, stress diseases have been treated mostly with tranquilizers, which often convert anxiety into depression.

An alternative to the use of tranquilizers is to learn self-control of anxiety and tension through progressive relaxation. Once a person learns progressive relaxation, he is often able to achieve for himself the beneficial effects of tranquilizing medications without experiencing their side effects. In 1929, Edmund Jacobson, an American physician, published his classic book *Progressive Relaxation,* in which he documented the effects of stress on body physiology and demonstrated that the regular practice of deep muscular relaxation was effective in restoring a healthy state of balance in bodily functions.

Progressive relaxation involves giving the patient careful instruction in first tensing and then relaxing many of the muscle groups throughout the body. The patient is told to pay careful attention to his feelings throughout this process. This technique is helpful in two respects: The patient learns what tension feels like in individual muscle groups and how the tension differs from relaxation; also, when proper instructions and suggestions are given, muscles tend to become more relaxed through this process. Deep relaxation slows heartbeat and respiration, raises skin temperature (an indication of emotional calmness), reduces stomach-acid production, decreases deep-tendon reflexes, and provides an increased sense of well-being. More recently, Herbert Benson has extensively studied relaxation techniques and has confirmed the physiological benefits of relaxation.

Autogenic Training. In 1932, J. H. Schultz published his first book on autogenic training, and during the next thirty-seven years, a great deal of clinical investigation showed the beneficial effects of this method. Autogenic training consists of a systematic mental focusing on short verbal phrases that suggest a state of autonomic balance. Patients are instructed to focus in a poised, alert way on six phrases:

My arms and legs are heavy.
My arms and legs are warm.
My heartbeat is calm and regular.
My breathing is relaxed and comfortable.
My abdomen is warm.
My forehead is cool.

Passive repetition of these phrases coupled with mental visualization of the desired goal lead to a 10 percent drop in pulse and blood pressure, an increase of one to two degrees in the skin temperature of hands and feet, better blood flow in abdominal organs, slowed breathing, decreased metabolic rate, slowed brain-wave activity, and a sense of well-being. By continuing to practice this technique, the patient has a release of emotional conflicts, improved performance, and less anxiety and tension. Improvement is seen in a consistent number of patients with a wide variety of psychosomatic or stress-related diseases.

Mental Training Exercises. Norman Shealy and others have used mental training exercises to teach patients with nerve damage how to improve their functioning. Many of their patients had failed to respond to surgery, drugs, or psychiatric treatment. The principle that guides much of their work is that if patients can be given feedback about how they are doing, they can learn to do better. For example, it is known that with proper practice of ear movements in front of a mirror, an individual can learn to voluntarily control his ear movements. In this case, visual feedback enhances the learning process. Similarly, individuals with partially damaged nerves that produce weak function of arms, face, bladder, or rectal sphincter can gain better muscular control by increasing the contraction of weak muscles.

In summary, by using a combined program of counseling with relaxation training, autogenic exercises, and biofeedback, it is possible to educate chronic-pain patients to successfully achieve the following therapeutic goals:

Reduce pain.
Stay off drugs.
Improve physical activity.
Avoid further surgery and hospitalization.

In chronic pain, as in most other stress-related disorders, most patients can be helped by proper training in self-regulation. The basic requirement seems to be that the patient continue to practice and to firmly *believe that a healthy, desired goal is possible.*

18

Three Alternatives to Surgery and Drugs in Pain Control

V. L. BRECKNER AND
T. FERRER-BRECKNER

IN THIS CHAPTER we will discuss three techniques of pain control that are available in this country today and do not involve the use of surgery or drugs. These methods are transcutaneous nerve stimulation, acupuncture, and nerve blocks.

They have the advantage of being less invasive than surgery and of leaving no potentially harmful scars. In contrast to the use of drugs, they do not cause addiction or affect brain alertness. In most cases, these treatments do not require hospitalization; they are therefore far less costly in terms of lost time and expenses. If complications occur and are properly handled, no permanent damage to any body organ or system is likely. There is no known risk of death with these techniques, and the chance of illness is minimal—nonexistent after a few hours.

Transcutaneous nerve stimulation. Electrical stimulation has been used as a method of pain control since the late nineteenth century. In that era a variety of stimulating machines was available. Such devices were popular in dental offices to relieve pain during drilling procedures and when pulling teeth. This method of pain relief later fell into disuse, mainly because of a lack of standardized procedures and equipment and because of wildly exaggerated claims on the part of some manufacturers.

More recently, electrical stimulation as a method of pain relief has been rediscovered. Surgical procedures in which electrodes were implanted in the dorsal section of the spinal cord began to be used in pain control. This rather formidable method of electrical stimulation is now losing popularity in favor of the more simplified electrodes placed on the skin. (The word *transcutaneous* means "outside the skin.")

Success with electrical stimulation has a good scientific basis. Large, fast-conducting nerve-fibers that have a thick coating of protective sheath (myelin) are much more easily stimulated by electrical current than are small, slow-conducting fibers that have no myelin coating. Physiologically, the large fibers are involved in the transmission of pleasant sensations, such as touch, grip, and stroking, as well as with unpleasant perceptions, such as pain.

It has been observed that while the large fibers are being electrically stimulated, a blockade against small-fiber pain-producing input is created at the spinal-cord level. Stimulating the large fibers seems to "shut the gate" on transmission of painful impulses. This is predicted in the "gate-control" theory, as we have noted earlier. Another factor that may be important in the use of stimulators is the simple effect of doing a procedure that causes an alteration in perceptions or in sensory input, distracting the patient from his habitual painful feelings. Whatever the mechanism, transcutaneous stimulators have become an important mainstay in the management of chronic pain.

The instruments themselves are fairly simple. They consist of a battery-operated device that generates a rapidly reappearing pulse of electrical current, of which there are two types. One presents an alternating current; its electrodes are not polarized. The second type has a direct current, and therefore the electrodes are polarized—either positive or negative. The instruments are small—about the size of a deck of cards—and can be carried by the patient in his own pocket. Electrodes can be taped to the skin in appropriate places and worn beneath clothing. The patient may stimulate himself at will during the day, thus supplying his own pain relief and making himself responsible for his own comfort.

Stimulator electrodes can be placed along the course of any nerve involved in the painful process. In the case of the alternating-current instrument, there is no difference between positive and negative electrodes in the placement along the nerve courses. However, in the direct-current instrument, the negative electrode should be put adjacent to the primary painful site. For instance, in cases of low-back pain with sciatic-nerve involvement, the negative electrode is placed over the back region, and the positive electrode is taped over the sciatic nerve along the back side of the painful leg. In cases of chronic pain from muscular disuse and fibrositis, the electrodes are simply placed over the affected muscles.

Experimentation is needed to find the ideal electrode placement. Sometimes this takes as long as a week of close cooperation between physician and patient. Repeated trials are also necessary in deciding what the correct wavelengths, frequencies, and voltages should be to achieve maximum effect.

The idea in using these instruments is to arouse the large fibers without stimulating the small fibers. To achieve this, the patient must be trained to recognize the maximum amount of electrical current capable of producing pleasant stimulation; if the stimulation becomes unpleasant, the goal is missed. Once the proper combinations have been worked out, the patient can rent one of these machines and take it to his own home; he can then work out a schedule of treatment that makes him comfortable throughout the day. Many people find that a fifteen-minute application early in the morning will result in markedly increased comfort for as long as four or five hours. Other people have to use the instrument more frequently.

Transcutaneous nerve stimulation is perhaps the least invasive of all physical methods of treatment. If properly used, muscle relaxation can be achieved, dilation of peripheral blood vessels noted, peripheral swelling reduced, and a marked improvement in comfort is frequently reported by the patient. From current information, nerve stimulation seems effective in a wide range of chronic-pain states—from back pain to phantom-limb pain, from various forms of neuropathies and neuralgias to those painful aftereffects of gunshot wounds known as causalgia. Transcutaneous nerve stimulation has the advantage of directly involving the patient in the treatment of his own problem. His degree of pain relief will be directly related to the amount of personal attention he devotes to applying the electrodes and using the device.

Acupuncture. This method was introduced into Western medicine during the past decade as a way to treat pain. Its philosophies and dogmas are complex, ethereal, and often incomprehensible to the Western mind. Although the reasons for its success are still obscure, it has been successful with a certain number of patients.

The treatment consists of inserting solid needles into specific sites of the patient's body. These sites are called acupuncture points and are exact locations diagrammed along longitudinal coordinates. Acupuncture points have no consistent relationship with human organ systems by the Western understanding of anatomy. However, there are certain generalities about acupuncture sites that should be noted.

Electrical resistance of the skin is consistently less over an acupuncture point than on the surrounding skin. By and large, patients whose comfort is improved by an acupuncture treatment will have no improvement in a later treatment if the needles are purposely placed close to, but not on, the exact acupuncture points, or if the acupuncture points are injected with local anesthesia first. In general, many acupuncture points are closely associated with places where nerves enter muscles (motor points) or where nerves come close to the surface of the skin.

It should be thoroughly understood that proper acupuncture is not a haphazard insertion of needles. It is an art in which precision of needle placement is vitally important. The acupuncture practitioner should not be casually trained; he must seriously pursue the learning of the art.

Nerve Blocks. A nerve block consists of introducing a hollow needle through the skin and directing it toward a nervous structure, such as a nerve trunk, nerve root, or sympathetic ganglion (nerve-relay point), which is supposedly involved in the patient's subjective experience of pain. Once the needle is correctly placed, an analgesic solution is injected that temporarily blocks the transmission of nerve impulses at the point of blockage. The duration of the nerve block is mainly contingent on the type of analgesic solution injected; the pain relief may vary from several hours with long-lasting solutions, such as Bupivacaine (Marcaine), to little more than one hour when procaine is used.

Understanding the rational use of nerve blocks depends on an appreciation of the anatomy involved. Essentially, there are two divisions of the peripheral nervous system: the somatic system and the automatic or autonomic system. The somatic system is essentially a system of conscious perception and control. Generally, the information we receive from the world about us comes via the somatic nervous system, which also controls our motor activities by way of impulses from the brain and spinal cord.

On the other hand, as we have noted earlier, the autonomic system controls functions that are not usually under conscious awareness, such as relaxation and contraction of blood vessels, production of sweat, secretion of various digestive enzymes in our intestinal tract, and the mobility of the intestine in carrying along food and digestive products.

Anatomically, these two systems, somatic and autonomic, are closely associated at many places in the same mixed nerve. At other places in the human body, however, the two systems are widely separated. It is therefore possible to inject an analgesic solution in an area that will affect only autonomic nerves.

According to the place in the body where the needle is placed, nerve blocks are subdivided into the following groups: (1) *spinal anesthesia,* in which the needle is inserted into the spinal canal, close to the nerve roots as they branch off the spinal cord; (2) *epidural anesthesia,* in which the needle is placed outside the spinal canal, between the outer, fibrous, protective sheath of the cord (the so-called dura-mater) and the inner side of the vertebrae within the bony vertebral column; (3) *somatic paravertebral blocks,* in which the needle is introduced close to the intervertebral foramen where the mixed nerve emerges from the spine (all mixed nerves from the cervical to the sacral region can be blocked by this route); (4) *peripheral nerve blocks,* in which a single nerve trunk is blocked along its course away from the spine (nerves that are often involved in painful experiences and that can be easily blocked peripherally are the trigeminal nerve—the main sensory nerve to the face—the intercostal nerves around the chest, and the sciatic nerve); (5) *sympathetic nerve blocks,* in which complete blockage of the autonomic sympathetic system can be achieved with three needles placed at the following levels: the seventh cervical vertebra in the neck (or the first thoracic vertebra in the back); the first lumbar vertebra; and the second or third lumbar vertebra in the low-back region. The needles are introduced as deep as a point close to the sympathetic ganglia, which are located bilaterally alongside the vertebral spine.

Western medicine has known the use of nerve blocks for pain control since the early twentieth century when the German surgeon Schlösser started experimenting with the blockage of nerves for treatment of conditions known as neuralgias, especially neuralgia of the trigeminal nerve. These techniques entered a new phase of promise after World Wars I and II, when numerous European and American scientists began using them in the diagnosis and therapy of visceral pain and other diseases.

Nerve blocks are still widely used to treat a variety of chronic-pain states. Good results, for example, can be expected in the treatment of low-back pain with injections of cortisone-like drugs in the spinal or epidural spaces, when irritation around the spinal nerve roots has occurred. Sympathetic blocks can also be useful in many cases of chronic back-pain and in a number of painful disorders of the limbs following various injuries, among which are causalgia and reflex sympathetic dystrophies. Excellent relief of upper-abdominal pain can be achieved with a block of the coeliac plexus, a network of autonomic nervous structures clustered in front of the first lumbar vertebra. Most of the painful impulses from the visceral organs in the upper part of the abdomen go through this plexus and can therefore be altered by blockage.

Another use of nerve blocks is to provide temporary pain-relief in an acute situation, allowing the patient to return to more normal function. An example of this would be a patient who has a series of fractured ribs and severe pain in his chest. Because of chest pain, he restricts his breathing and is reluctant to cough. This can result in lung collapse from accumulated secretions. Nerve blocks in this situation will dramatically change the patient's condition. For several hours, he will be able to cough and breathe deeply and bring up secretions that are causing his problem.

Nerve blocks are by no means a noninvasive therapy. Central-nervous-system reaction to local anesthetics may occur, causing convulsions, breathing difficulties, and cardiovascular collapse. Allergic reactions and various minor complications at the site of introduction of the needle have also been reported. It should be noted that all serious complications from nerve blocks occur within 15–30 minutes; it is therefore imperative for doctors to keep a patient under observation for at least half an hour following treatment. It is also mandatory that the physician performing the block be well trained in advanced life-support technology and have all equipment for cardiorespiratory resuscitation promptly available.

Little is really known about the exact mechanism by which pain relief is achieved using these methods. Nerve blocks (mostly sympathetic nerve-blocks) and electrical stimulation have in common the properties of altering sensory inputs and increasing blood flow in the area that has been blocked or electrically stimulated. It is conceivable that altered sensory inputs reduce the sufferer's perception of whatever he has learned to feel as painful. Increased blood circulation in disused muscles and visceral organs may also help induce a return to normal functions.

These mechanisms may explain why nerve blocks, while lasting only a few hours, occasionally provide days and weeks of subjective comfort. However, it must be recognized that no treatment by itself can be fully successful unless it is structured in comprehensive management programs involving physical reeducation, emotional readjustment, and correction of drug abuse.

19

Common Painful Experiences: Headaches

S. F. BRENA

HEADACHE IS ONE OF our oldest recorded diseases. Easily recognizable symptoms of migraine headache are described in almost every historical medical text.

The pre-Columbian Incas of Peru apparently drilled holes into the skull to relieve the agony of severe headaches. We infer this from skulls unearthed along the shores of Lake Titicaca, some with evidence of healed burr-holes. Medieval doctors in Europe also used skull-surgery and bloodletting as a therapy for headache, along with a few drugs, mostly cathartics.

Studies in anatomy and physiology during the Italian Renaissance and the modern age have brought an end to such crude and often deadly techniques for the relief of headaches, but we are not dramatically more advanced in our methods of treatment of this age-old pain problem.

Even today we are far from having a clear and satisfactory understanding of all headache phenomena, and therefore modern headache therapy remains empirical, although based on sound scientific principles.

Under the label "headache" a variety of health problems are bound together, so that headache can be viewed either as a symptom of various diseases or as a state of disease itself. It is estimated that at least 10 percent of all Americans suffer periodic headaches; twelve million of these are severely handicapped by migraine.

There are two broad categories of headache:

Headache as a symptom of disease. A steady, constant, deep, throbbing headache of recent onset suggests the presence of a potentially deadly disease, such as brain tumor, aneurysm, high blood-pressure, toxic states from liver or kidney failure, encephalitis, brain abscess, or other intracranial (inside-the-skull) infection.

Headache as a disease: migraine and tension headache. A general way to differentiate between headache as a symptom and as a disease is by its frequency rate. Migraine and tension headaches usually come and go with various degrees of frequency and intensity. Attacks may last for hours or days, then fade away, leaving the patient free of pain. Both migraine and tension headache can become major health problems, like any other chronic-pain state, through the sick-behavior learning process and related social interactions.

It is not easy in every case to tell the difference between tension headache and migraine. Migraine is typically viewed today as a vascular disorder in which an increase of blood flowing through pain-sensitive blood vessels helps sustain the discomfort. Migraine attacks are usually paired with loss of appetite, nausea, and vomiting. They often are associated with sensory, mood, or motor disturbances. Migraine seems to run in families. In the last decade, research has suggested that migraine headache may be triggered by the formation of inflammatory substances around the arteries and veins of the skull. Five or more groups of these substances seem associated with migraine attacks: catecholamines, histamine, serotonin, peptide kinins, and prostaglandins. All of these substances appear to play a role in the process of vascular inflammation that leads to a migraine attack.

Tyramine, a chemical found in high concentration in cheeses and strong beers, can evoke migraine in some subjects. Tyramine is also formed in the intestines by the bacterial transformation of the amino acid called tyrosine, a chemical forerunner of the catecholamines epinephrine and norepinephrine. The human body quickly deactivates tyramine with proper enzyme action; however, a defect in the metabolic disposal of this chemical may lead to high blood-concentrations of tyramine. Such a defect has been reported in some migraine patients, thus linking migraine to a possible genetic deficiency as well as to certain foods or drink.

A unified theory of migraine recently has been proposed to account for all phenomena in a migraine attack. Following various physical and emotional stresses, a change in vascular activity occurs within the arteries and veins at the base of the brain and in the meningeal vessels in the brain's lining. An initial painless constriction of these vessels leads to reduction of blood flow to the brain, with a decreased supply of oxygen and related local metabolic disturbance. This initial phase is usually followed by a dilation of arteries inside and outside the skull, bringing a greater blood flow to the brain and brain edema (swelling). This change in the skull vessels provokes the formation of active or inflammatory substances, as mentioned above; a pounding ache in the head is thus generated.

Migraine headache, then, might be described as a transient, relatively benign biological storm, produced by the interactions of the central and peripheral autonomic nervous systems and by contraction and expansion of blood vessels inside and outside the skull. There is also vascular inflammation.

In contrast to migraine, tension headache is primarily a muscular disorder, often sustained by an underlying degenerative osteoarthritis in the upper vertebral region or in the jaw joint. (*Osteo* means "bone.") Typically, the victim complains of recurring headaches that vary in frequency and severity and often start in the back of the head and neck, spreading toward the top of the head and frontal area. Some patients describe a tension headache as a "constricting band" tightened around the whole of their head. By feeling the head, a physician may discover several tender points over the entire scalp and at the rear of the head and neck, often all the way down the back of the neck to the shoulders and thoracic back region.

Tension headaches in this form are likely to be the equivalent of low-back pain: Chronic irritation of the upper cervical (neck) nerve roots by a process of degenerative, spinal osteoarthritis triggers and sustains various muscular disorders, with related discomfort. The end product of prolonged muscular dysfunction is probably similar to that of blood-vessel abnormalities. The muscles involved undergo metabolic derangements: They swell with fluid and show abnormal concentrations of lactic acid and possibly other irritants (peptide kinins, histamine, serotonin), which accumulate locally and further upset blood flow to the muscles and muscle metabolism.

A common pattern is thus set in which tension headache develops into a full-blown migraine attack.

Most textbooks and medical articles on headache emphasize emotional factors in tension and migraine headaches. No doubt, personality and emotional problems are sometimes converted into headache symptoms; for example, a person who is a hypochondriac will often have a headache. However, I disagree with the view that artificially puts vascular, tension, and "psychogenic" headaches into different categories.

Mind and body cannot be separated. Emotional tension can be converted into muscular tension, while inversely a muscular disorder—or any other bodily disorder—can easily produce an emotional derangement. The two problems reinforce each other and often lead to vascular complications, ultimately to a dreaded migraine attack.

Once the pattern is set and headache episodes repeat themselves with increasing frequency and intensity, a "breaking point" is reached where the balance of well-being is upset. The patient becomes increasingly unbalanced, obsessed by fear of a migraine attack, dysfunctional, depressed, cries out for relief at any cost, and winds up with multiple-drug abuse and complications. He is soon crippled by the Five D's syndrome.

Migraine headache responds well to drugs that contain a chemical called ergot. Such preparations may help prevent the changes in blood flow in cerebral vessels that are known to lay the ground for migraine attacks. However, the ergot drugs are dangerous because of their side effects and should never be taken without careful supervision of a physician.

Abuse of ergot preparations induces a condition known as ergotism, which is also seen in patients poisoned by contaminated rye. Ergotism is manifested by nausea, vomiting, coldness and cramps in the arms and legs, and increased intracranial pressure. This pressure inside the skull causes more headache and may prompt the uninformed patient to take more drugs. This is particularly dangerous in the case of women on contraceptive medication who suffer from exacerbation of headaches while taking the hormones. Those who ingest large quantities of ergot drugs may get increased brain pressure and a cerebral "stroke."

Both migraine (at early onset) and tension headaches respond well to preparations containing aspirin, which seems the drug of choice in such cases. In most of the commonly sold drugs for headache problems, however, aspirin is combined with phenacetin and caffeine. Such combinations actually increase the risk of side effects in cases of drug abuse. Most dangerous are compounds labeled as "specific" for headache relief—preparations containing codeine and a barbiturate in addition to the combination aspirin-phenacetin-caffeine, in which the habit-forming effects of an opiate and a barbiturate are added to the toxic side effects of aspirin and phenacetin in cases of drug abuse.

In recent years a trend toward long-term management of headache problems has developed. Rather than poisoning the patient with drugs, better results are achieved by going to the root of the problem and teaching the patient how to control the muscular and vascular abnormalities that seem to trigger painful episodes. Studies are underway in this area and promising results have been reported along these lines: (1) training the patient to relax particular groups of muscles voluntarily by practicing appropriate relaxation exercises; (2) training the patient to relax particular groups of muscles with muscle biofeedback techniques; (3) training the migraine patient to shift the flow of blood from brain to limbs with thermal (heat) biofeedback.

In cases where relaxation training and drug therapy fail to produce satisfactory results, psychotherapy should be considered in an effort to resolve unconscious emotional conflicts and personality maladjustments, so that corresponding physical tension can be relaxed. Actually, psychotherapy should not be confined to headache problems only; it may be helpful in most cases of chronic pain that fail to respond to conservative reeducational programs, where deep-rooted and maladjusted emotional forces interact and perpetuate physical distress.

20

Common Painful Experiences: Low-Back Pain

J. R. DE ANDRADE

SOMETIME IN THEIR active lives, 80 percent of all humans will have low-back pain. Men are as afflicted as often as women, white-collar workers as often as blue-collar workers. Recent studies in the United States and Sweden have shown that low-back pain is the single most costly ailment in the 30–60 age group.

Low-back pain can be triggered by a wide variety of organic disorders, most of them in the spinal column but some outside the spine. Diseases of the lower abdominal organs, especially ailments in the pelvic cavity, such as those affecting the female organs, are frequent causes of low-back pain. Backaches can also be found in connection with kidney disease, and more rarely, tumors of the spinal cord and spinal roots. Organs in the upper part of the abdomen, such as the stomach and liver, may cause backache higher up in the spine.

By far the most common place of origin of low-back pain is the skeletal structures of the spine. Fractures and infections of the vertebral column are always accompanied by severe, acute back pain, but these are not frequent. On the other hand, the so-called lumbar-disc syndrome is the single most widespread vertebral disorder causing acute pain, which in some circumstances becomes chronic. Other names for lumbar-disc syndrome are spondylosis, collapsed intravertebral disc, lumbago, and sciatica.

To understand the causes and treatment of low-back pain, it is helpful to know some basic things about the anatomy of the vertebral column and the spinal cord.

The vertebral column, or spine, is made up of twenty-six or twenty-seven vertebrae. Each vertebra has a body and three sets of processes—bony protuberances that afford a union with the vertebrae above and below. Behind the vertebral bodies is a spinal canal that contains the spinal cord and roots of the spinal nerves. There are seven neck or cervical vertebrae, twelve chest or thoracic vertebrae, five low-back or lumbar vertebrae, one sacral piece (the sacrum), and one or two tailbone (coccygeal) segments.

The vertebrae are arranged in the form of a column that supports the body and allows movement while protecting the spinal cord. Between each vertebra is a space called the intervertebral foramen; it is here that the spinal nerves emerge from the spinal canal, one pair of nerves for each vertebral segment. To allow movement, there are two sets of joints in the spine; these are the disc joints and posterior joints.

The disc joints are between the vertebral bodies. Each disc is composed of a soft center (nucleus pulposus) and a fibrous tissue ring (annulus fibrosus). The disc joint gives the spine great shock-absorbing powers, with the soft center acting as a fluid ball-bearing within constraints of the fibrous-tissue ring. Posterior joints are located between the bony protuberances of two adjacent vertebrae; they are constructed in a manner similar to other movable joints, such as the knee.

The vertebrae are kept together by a thick feltwork of fibrous tissue called ligaments, and by various groups of muscles called paraspinal muscles, whose main function is to straighten out the spine after it has bent forward. Interestingly, there are no spinal muscles that bend the spine forward; this function is performed by the muscles of the abdomen.

The spinal cord runs down the spinal canal from the base of the skull to the first lumbar vertebra, which is located approximately at the level of the lower end of the ribs. The cord is made up of nerve cells, nerve fibers, and supporting tissue that holds the cells and fibers together. Various nerve pathways that carry pain-producing impulses run up the spinal cord toward the brain from all the spinal segments.

The spinal cord gives off one pair of spinal nerves for each vertebral segment. There are thirty-one or thirty-two pairs of spinal nerves, including eight in the neck, twelve in the chest, five low-back, five sacral (buttocks), and one or two in the tailbone. Each spinal nerve has an anterior, motor, root and a posterior, sensory root.

Pain-producing impulses travel along both the large- and small-fiber nerve-networks of the body and reach the spinal cord via the posterior (rear) sensory roots. Both roots join to form a mixed sensory-motor spinal nerve, which, as it emerges from the spine, gives off a posterior branch that supplies the back muscles near the vertebrae.

When this nerve branch is irritated or pinched by narrowing of the vertebral foramen, it often causes low-back pain.

Spinal nerves frequently involved in the experience of low-back pain are the sciatic and femoral nerves. The sciatic nerve runs down the back of the thigh and leg to the foot, while the femoral nerve travels down the front of the thigh and leg.

The entire spinal cord is covered by various protective membranes, which are similar to the meningeal linings of the brain. Both the brain and the spinal cord are sheltered from concussion by the presence of a clear, water-like fluid called the cerebral-spinal fluid. Between the outer spinal-cord membrane and the bone of the vertebrae there is a space, called the epidural space, which is filled with fat and blood vessels that lead to and from the cord. This space is crossed by the spinal nerves on their way out.

The vertebral column has several vitally important life functions, including (1) housing and protecting the spinal cord and its nervous elements, (2) forming a base of support for the trunk and transmitting force from the head and upper part of the body to the pelvis, and (3) allowing movement that involves the action of muscles.

The precise cause of pain in lumbar-disc syndrome is not known. The spine's feltwork of fibrous tissue is well supplied with nerves, and irritation of these nerves may generate painful impulses. Also, the lumbar disc can be displaced backward, thus pressing on the nerves and causing discomfort. The disc may bulge out or the soft center may rupture, allowing a fragment of the softer material to protrude backward.

When only the low-back area is painful, the disc is probably involved without pressure on nerve roots. When pain shoots down along the sciatic nerve, the disc is likely to be pressing on sciatic-nerve roots. Pain is sometimes perceived in the buttocks because the nerves that supply the lumbar discs serve the skin of the buttocks as well. It should be remembered that disc pressure on a nerve is painful because the nerve is confined in a small space and cannot move out of the way.

Factors leading to disc problems include aging, osteoarthritis of the joints of the spine, and stress forces on the vertebral discs.

As a person ages, the soft centers of the discs get drier and more brittle and the fibrous rings grow stiffer. The soft centers become less like bags of fluid and more like bags of jelly full of fruit and pits. All the fibrous tissue in the body, including the fibrous ring, is more brittle and is subject to rupture more readily.

Osteoarthritis is a wear-and-tear disease of the joints that is also aggravated by aging. It affects moving joints such as the posterior joints of the spine. If the spine is involved and joint cartilage is lost, the joint collapses, perhaps to a very small degree, such as two or three millimeters. This, together with the collapse of the disc, causes the vertebrae to come closer together. One result is that the nerve root emerging from the spinal cord is rather tightly confined, so if any further source of pressure arises, such as a bulging or herniated disc, the nerve root will sustain excessive pressure.

In regard to stresses on the disc, it must be remembered that these are often greater than mere body weight. Lever forces greatly magnify disc stress. If we consider the disc a fulcrum, and a force of one hundred pounds acts ten inches in front of the disc, the result is a force of one thousand inch-pounds. If the balancing force is two inches behind the disc, then five hundred pounds of force would have to be exerted to achieve a thousand-pound balance. This five hundred pounds plus the original one hundred would mean six hundred pounds are exerted on the disc. Considerably larger forces are exerted dynamically when a weight is suddenly lifted or the individual jumps from a height.

As the intervertebral spaces narrow and pressure builds on nerve roots, critical changes occur in the blood supply to the roots themselves. Each nerve root carries its own blood supply as a fine network of small arteries and veins on the outside of the root. Pressure slightly above normal may collapse these small vessels, resulting in congestion and swelling.

Swelling inside the rigid wall of the intervertebral space further increases pressure on the nerve root. Nerve-root irritation leads to muscle tension with its own metabolic upset. Electromyographic studies have shown functional derangement of spinal muscles in patients suffering from low-back pain. Pain relief and reeducation may help bring a return to normal.

Usually, lumbar-disc syndrome starts with an episode of physical stress, but in most cases this is minor. For example, simple bending or picking up a handkerchief may trigger the symptoms. Lifting a heavy weight can also do it. It should be remembered that even simple bending produces a lot of force on vertebral discs. Pain may occur immediately after the stress or it may develop gradually over the course of the next few days. Pain that develops immediately is probably due to the disc physically irritating the nerves; when the onset of pain is delayed, it probably signifies that the injured structure has become inflamed and is now irritating the nerves. In some cases, multiple episodes of stress are required before clinical back-pain occurs. Discomfort may be represented by a feeling of uneasiness in the back for several days and also by stiffness.

Lumbar-disc syndrome is seen in various manifestations. There is a difference between the episodic, acute form of this musculoskeletal disorder and its occurrence as chronic pain. The acute type is a minor emergency and requires prompt bed rest, which usually brings a remission of symptoms. An acute episode of lumbago or sciatica is often followed by recurrent episodes of semiacute pain; between attacks, however, patients may be completely pain-free or may experience various degrees of aching and stiffness in the back.

On the other hand, chronic disc-syndrome involves additional problems, which are probably sustained by emotional arousal, the breaking down of inhibitory brain activity, and the learning processes of chronic illness, along with other mechanisms. The patient with chronic disc-syndrome often undergoes multiple surgical procedures in an effort to find relief.

Generally, most forms of acute and semiacute low-back pain are relieved by bed rest, which decreases disc strain and prevents aggravation. In time, the bulging protrusion or herniation will scar down and shrink, thus relieving the discomfort. Bed rest may be usefully supplemented with vertebral traction. This can be applied lightly and continuously to maintain rest in a selected posture, or it can be used heavily and intermittently in an attempt to actually separate the vertebrae, minimize the bulging of the disc, and open the intervertebral spaces.

Physical exercise can help in strengthening muscles and in mobilization of a stiff spine. There are various combinations of flexion and extension exercises—the best-known are the Williams exercises. Flexion exercises are beneficial to the posterior vertebral structures and help open up the intervertebral spaces. Extension exercises jam together the posterior spine structures but tend to relieve pressure on the disc.

Exercises should be matched by proper relaxation training between exercises. In chronic back-pain a great deal of discomfort is caused by reactive tightening of various muscle groups, causing in itself much painful stimulation. The Jacobson relaxation technique, muscle biofeedback, and Transcendental Meditation are useful tools in training chronic low-back sufferers to relax efficiently. Exercises and relaxation techniques that are practiced today for low-back pain relief have been recommended for centuries in the teaching of Hatha Yoga.

Since lumbar-disc syndrome involves pressure relationships among disc, intervertebral spaces, posterior joints of the spine, and nerve roots, positional changes among these structures may result in improvement. This type of management forms the main basis of therapy in osteopathy and chiropractic. Mobilization medicine is a legitimate field of modern medicine, and in some cases it helps bring relief. The techniques vary so widely that it is not practical here to describe them, but generally they involve some form of traction to separate the bones, usually by taking advantage of the upper and lower extremities to act as levers. Discs and posterior joints are then led gently but firmly through a full range of motion and a little bit beyond.

Rest and immobility relieve low-back pain, so it would appear that immobilization in a cast or brace would have some benefit. However, even with immobilization, considerable force is passed through the spine that cannot be counteracted by a brace or cast. Also, because of the soft tissue around the torso and the depth of the spine, it is impossible to truly immobilize this area. Another problem is that immobilization results in disuse of muscles. What is needed is to give the patient the ability to transfer force away from the spine, often through the agency of muscles; hence, a brace or cast should rarely be used.

Three types of surgery may be done to relieve low-back pain: removal of the herniated disc, vertebral fusion, and nerve severance. The results of disc removal are good if the offending disc is correctly identified and successfully removed and the spine is otherwise in good shape. But when irreversible osteoarthritic changes in the spine are present, simple removal of the disc is not enough to relieve pain; in these cases, a fusion may be advisable. This procedure consists of putting a bone graft between the vertebrae so as to make two adjacent vertebrae one bone by solid, bony bridging; it eliminates movement between the fused structures. Spinal fusion, however, is a difficult operation and not always successful. Nerve severance for relief of back pain has been abandoned by most neurosurgeons, because it provides incomplete and only temporary pain relief with a risk of serious complications, including an actual increase of burning pain in the legs, often described as much worse than the original back or sciatic pain.

Nerve blocks, as we have noted, are effective ways to relieve both acute and chronic back-pain. For the most part, epidural and sympathetic blocks are used. In addition to a local anesthetic, cortisone is often injected. Cortisone prevents inflammation and tends to relieve the swelling that follows; it is thus a useful addition. Theoretically, these injections should last no more than several hours. For some unknown reason, however, pain relief is often longer and may be permanent, as we've mentioned.

21

Common Painful Experiences: Chest Pain

W. D. HAMMONDS

TO JOE C., CHEST PAIN came as a terrifying experience. He was immediately certain it was heart disease, the leading killer of American men. Through media information on heart disease, Joe had picked up the term *angina pectoris,* and now it was like a menacing sword to him.

The fact that Joe is a fifty-year-old executive who is overweight and smokes at least two packs of cigarettes a day—a man who delights in eating cholesterol-rich foods and doesn't get much exercise—gives him every right to be afraid. Largely because of his own habits, he is in a high-risk category for heart trouble.

Angina pectoris is an attack of chest pain produced by insufficient blood flow to the heart muscle through narrowed, diseased coronary arteries. The disease is sometimes called ischemic heart pain, meaning a painful disorder produced by poor oxygen supply to the heart because of impaired arterial blood flow.

William Heberdeen was the first to describe the symptoms of angina pectoris in his *Commentaries on the History and Cure of Disease,* in 1802. His description is remarkable for its completeness, considering when it was written. Heberdeen mentioned all the important features of an attack: onset following a physical effort or emotional distress, more common in men over fifty, relieved by rest, pain begins in midchest and radiates to left arm, often fatal.

Associating chest pain radiating to the left arm with heart disease has empirical roots that can be traced back to folk medicine. It often causes anxiety and fear in people who may have learned about this symptom from friends or relatives who actually experienced an episode of ischemic heart pain.

In fact, chest pain radiating to the left arm does not necessarily signal heart trouble. Any disorder of the deep structures of the upper chest can cause such an experience. The intensity of chest pain is also not related to the seriousness of the underlying problem. The most trivial medical ailment can give rise to severe pain, whereas potentially lethal disorders, including cancer of the lungs, can be painless almost to the end of their natural course.

The heart is among the least frequent of all the possible causes of chest pain; cancer and infectious lung diseases also do not often cause great discomfort in the chest. On the other hand, muscles and bony skeletal structures are among the most common causes of chest pain. (In Joe C.'s case, the pain problem involved chest muscles, but not his heart.)

The chest is a well-muscled structure. Powerful muscle

groups from the abdomen, arms, and neck are attached to the chest wall, and there are three layers of muscles in spaces between the ribs. Chest muscles receive their nerve supply from nerve roots located both in the cervical (neck) and dorsal (mid-back) segments of the spinal cord. Osteoarthritis involves degenerative changes in the vertebral bony and joint structures. These changes cause a narrowing of the intervertebral spaces and may result in chronic irritation of nerve roots, with related muscular irritability and tension that is perceived as chest discomfort. (This process is described in the previous chapter.)

Degenerative vertebral changes are most frequent in the neck area of the spine, due to the wide range of motion that takes place at this level because of head and shoulder movements. Osteoarthritis is less frequent in the dorsal segment, since it is relatively well protected against wear-and-tear by the rib cage, which limits vertebral motion. Nerve-root irritation triggers waves of painful impulses that are perceived as a deep, boring, aching discomfort with occasional sharp piercing pain of a "lightning" character when a sensory root is pinched.

It is this sharp or lightning-type chest pain that often triggers a high level of anxiety and fear of a heart attack. Fear causes an outpouring of adrenalin into the blood stream, with related changes in blood pressure and muscular function. Sustained muscular tension produces metabolic derangement in the muscles, resulting in fibrositis, a painful swelling of disused muscles. Also, changes in blood pressure disturb the patient with feelings of choking, pounding in chest and neck, and occasional headaches. A cycle is thus generated in which chest pain from a trivial nerve-root irritation produces emotional arousal and physiological changes, which in turn further upset the patient and perpetuate the painful experience.

Among the most common fibrositis syndromes are those involving the pectoral muscles of the chest and the large trapezius muscles that attach onto the occipital (rear) region of the skull and all along the cervical and dorsal vertebral column. Dysfunction and disuse in these two muscle groups, both of which receive their nerve supply from cervical nerve-roots, may cause headaches, chest pain, and upper-back pains. Relatives of patients who have recently suffered heart attacks are prone to develop muscular chest pain from vicarious symptoms related to learning and concern about their sick kin. Treatment of chest pain from osteoarthritis and fibrositis is the same as for other forms of skeletal and muscular disorders.

Less-common causes of chest pain are the various disorders involving the intercostal nerves of the rib cage. The ribs themselves are rather exposed to injury and may be broken or dislodged from their joints, which connect with the sternum (breastbone). Excruciating pain, decrease in respiratory movements of the rib cage, and a high risk of pulmonary complications often follow. A fairly common damage to nervous structures is the one produced by "shingles," or herpes zoster, a viral infection of nerves with high incidence on intercostal (rib cage) nerves. The herpetic infection is sustained by the same virus that causes chicken-pox in children; it occurs most often in the elderly or chronically ill but can happen also in young and healthy individuals.

In its early stage, shingles is marked by a rash of pustules distributed along the course of one or more intercostal nerves around the chest. The rash is accompanied by a burning type of pain that can be quite severe, waxing and waning in paroxysms. After one or two weeks, the rash goes away and the acute pain disappears in all but a small percentage of people.

Why some patients who have suffered a herpes zoster infection develop chronic, burning pain along the strip of skin touched by the rash is not known. It is tempting to speculate that these unfortunate individuals fit the profile of pain-prone people because of some preexisting personality maladjustment. No study thus far has documented such a relationship, however.

Pain from postherpetic nerve damage can be relieved by a combination of physical therapy—including massages, the intermittent use of a hand vibrator over the painful area, and ice packs—and a few selected drugs, such as phenothiazines (Prolixin), antidepressants (Elavil), and other drugs, such as Tegretol. A less common but similar nerve damage that produces chest pain is caused by injury to intercostal nerves during open-chest surgery. This well-known medically induced complication is a painful experience similar to the discomfort of postherpetic neuralgia, and occasionally it responds to the same treatment.

A poorly known and rather trivial pain syndrome that mimics a heart attack is the so-called Tietze's syndrome. It is actually a painful swelling of the junction between ribs and cartilage in the front of the chest, close to the breastbone. This problem is also called anterior-chest syndrome and is believed to be caused by repeated pressure on the anterior (front) chest wall from faulty posture and working conditions that require leaning over a bench at chest level. Though the pain is disturbing at the time, the syndrome is self-limiting and needs no treatment in a large proportion of individuals suffering from it. Occasionally, when a pain-prone person is affected by Tietze's syndrome, the mild pain-experience becomes a major distress factor with activation of learned pain, drug misuse, and self-perpetuating suffering well in excess of its physical origin.

Harmful stimulation in any of the organ systems located inside the rib cage, in the biliary tracts of the liver, or in the diaphragm (a muscle located between the thorax and the abdomen) can be perceived as chest pain. Acute chest pain may be associated with lung infections or lung collapse, with myocardial infarction (heart attack), acute pericarditis (inflammation of the sac that contains the heart), or with aneurysms tearing on the walls of the aorta (great artery of the heart). It may also be the only symptom of a hernia of the esophagus, an inflammation of the gall bladder, or pleurisy.

It is up to the diagnostic acumen of the physician and to an astute use of laboratory and radiologic studies to determine whether acute chest pain has a cardiac origin, comes from other visceral sources, or is related to muscle or nerve disorders. The task is not easy and often taxes the diagnostic skills of the practitioner. For instance, acute gall-bladder disease can cause left-anterior chest pain and severe discomfort behind the breastbone, closely resembling the pain from an ischemic heart condition or myocardial infarction.

Consideration of the fiber pathways that carry pain impulses to the central nervous system helps throw some light on the often-puzzling characteristic of chest pain from so many different organ systems and neuromuscular structures. For example, some of the small fibers from the heart pass through sympathetic ganglia (nerve relays) in the upper chest. Nerve fibers to the skin and muscles of the mid- and upper-chest as well as nerve fibers to the arms also pass through the same ganglia. Meanwhile, other fibers from the heart go through sympathetic ganglia in the neck, where nerve fibers to the face also cross. This crossover of various fiber networks at the ganglia switchboard shows how heart-attack pain can travel to the arms, neck, and jaw. Common nerve pathways and ganglia crossovers are shared by all internal organs of the chest, which explains why the experience of pain from such organs has the same quality whether it originates in the lungs, heart, or esophagus.

If the causes of *acute* chest pain are difficult to separate, *chronic* chest pain is even harder to deal with once an emotional arousal has clouded the picture. Patients who complain of chronic chest pain from minor muscular involvements often get unpredictable relief following curious rituals, such as the use of poultices, plasters, massages, and acupuncture. Surprisingly, patients with actual chronic heart-disease may get some relief of chest pain from these placebo-like treatments.

One explanation for the placebo response in patients who have suffered a myocardial infarction is the high level of anxiety and death fear in these chronic sufferers. They become so abnormally aware of sensory experiences in their chests that even minor changes in sensation may be interpreted as either pain relief or pain increase. Both sham operations and surgery designed to improve the heart's blood supply have been shown to be equally effective in relieving the pain of intractable angina pectoris. Nerve blocks at various sites of the chest will often relieve chronic chest pain in patients with heart disease. Both surgery and nerve blocks cause sensory changes by cutting or blocking the fibers of sensory nerves; a changed pattern of sensory inputs may be enough to reassure the patient, decrease his anxiety temporarily, and release his tension in a feeling of pain relief.

Chest pain is a baffling problem. In its acute form, it fully justifies a comprehensive medical investigation by the cautious physician. In its chronic form, however, chest pain calls for restraint, competence, and wisdom to avoid repetitive medical work-ups that may result in nothing more than sending the patient's anxiety and fear skyrocketing.

Appropriate drugs in dealing with documented causes of acute chest pain are essential to bring the problem under control and eventually cure it, if possible. But the indiscriminate use of opiates and tranquilizers in chronic chest pain of dubious origin will only add an addiction problem to a patient's pain-related dysfunction.

In the treatment of patients recovering from myocardial infarctions (heart attacks), long periods of bed rest and immobility once were prescribed. This created many complications, which further taxed the patient's recovery. Additional heart attacks were sometimes noted when patients tried to become active again following long bed-rest.

But recently, a different type of cardiac rehabilitation program has been engineered for patients recovering from myocardial infarction. As soon as the acute heart-episode is over, patients now are structured in a careful program of daily increasing activities under close medical supervision. They are rehabilitated to function as closely as possible to normal and as soon as they can, relative to the severity of their heart disease.

22

Common Painful Experiences: Pain and Sexual Function

I. P. UNIKEL

PHYSICIANS OFTEN SEE a pattern of reduced sexual activity in patients with chronic pain. Poor sexual performance can put extra stress on already overburdened marriages, adding to feelings of inadequacy and helplessness in the chronic sufferer.

Many factors are involved in making sexual behavior unsatisfactory. For example, the heavy and continuing use of opiates can depress the central nervous system and bring a decrease in sexual interest. Barbiturates, sedatives, and the excessive use of alcohol can have a similar effect. In a more direct fashion, opiates can produce a lessened capacity for sexual performance. A male who is on high doses of such medications may have trouble producing a good erection, or will quickly lose it. Because patients with chronic pain often abuse depressant drugs, they are candidates for diminished sexuality as a result.

Mr. and Mrs. John R. are an example of this problem. Their domestic differences have caused them to quarrel, but instead of trying to reach a compromise, John decides to avoid intercourse with his wife, in an effort to make her submit to his authority. The project misfires; the wife seems unconcerned, and John soon is frustrated by his voluntary sexual deprivation. He becomes restless, cannot sleep, and goes to his family physician for counseling.

The doctor finds nothing physically wrong but notes the symptoms of anxiety. For lack of anything better, he prescribes Valium, one five-milligram tablet at bedtime. For a while things seem to quiet down, but as drug-habituation grows, the one tablet at bedtime becomes two and then four, six, eight each day. Soon John finds himself less sexually capable than he used to be; he is having erection problems and a lot of "muscle spasms" when his body is low on Valium. He is also more confused and less able to cope with his marital problems.

One or more of the following disasters are bound to happen: John's wife will seek divorce on grounds of mental anguish and sexual deprivation; he will lose his job because of growing inefficiency; he will have an accident because of poor performance and poor judgment caused by drug abuse.

Emotional problems, such as anxiety and depression, can also lead to sexual abstinence. Studies have shown that sexuality is often diminished by various physical disorders, including those involving the sexual organs and reproductive system, diabetes, multiple sclerosis, and other chronic diseases. In fact, a decrease in libido, impotence in males, or frigidity in females may be an early alarm that something is wrong.

Apart from generalized diseases, a number of localized disorders, such as hip-joint arthritis and lumbar-disc disease, may lead to discomfort when the sufferer engages in sexual intercourse. Such problems can therefore be a major cause of sexual malfunction. Pain associated with sexual activity is also a frequent complaint of patients who have undergone multiple surgeries in the lower abdomen or low-back area.

Masters and Johnson recommend a careful evaluation of all physical and emotional factors involved in cases of women who have painful intercourse. They emphasize three main physical indicators: relationship between anatomical location and pain description, severity of pain, and the timing of pain during intercourse. Such physical disorders as bacterial infections of the vagina or vaginal sensitivity to the rubber in diaphragms and to other substances, including soaps, may exist.

Inadequate lubrication of the vagina may be a result of the thinning of vaginal walls caused by lessened hormone production as part of the aging process. However, failure to lubricate is also related to diminished sexual arousal and may be reflected in the woman's negative attitude toward sex in general and toward her sexual partner in particular. Indeed, Masters and Johnson consider vaginal lubrication to be the female counterpart of penile erection in the male.

The matter becomes even more complicated when people who are aging or are otherwise physically infirm begin to worry about their sexual adequacy. Anxiety can only make their condition worse. A woman's anxiety about her own or her partner's inadequacy will also inhibit lubrication of the vagina; the same will happen when the woman is worried about getting pregnant.

Fear of pain can have similar effects. The usual symptoms of painful intercourse that are primarily physiological are itching, burning, and aching. According to Masters and Johnson, women who imagine or contrive pain to avoid intercourse do not tend to report these symptoms. These women usually describe their pain as "a hurting deep in the vagina during thrusting."

Sexual behaviors are learned and reinforced by their own consequences. They often display a tendency to closely interact with sick behaviors. An example of this is one in which a person exaggerates pain complaints to avoid sexual intercourse with a partner whom he or she subconsciously dislikes and wishes to see hurt. The main drawback of such avoidance behavior is that it persists long after the need for it has passed. The individual may continue staying away from desirable as well as undesirable activity.

Two examples of sexual avoidance, taken from actual case records, will illustrate some of the points made above.

Mary S. has a mild case of multiple sclerosis and develops a bladder defect with some inconvenience during sexual intercourse or while sitting. She becomes obsessed by the fear of wetting her clothes in public or while enjoying sex with her husband. Her obsession impairs her sexual and social activities and produces a state of profound depression. One day she slips and falls on the floor of her kitchen and hurts her tailbone. Under normal circumstances, this minor injury would be over and forgotten in a few days, but not in Mary's case.

She now has a true case of coccygodynia, or tailbone pain, which justifies her avoidance of sex. Moreover, she has a socially acceptable excuse to get up from her chair while socializing to "get relief from pain." Actually, she uses this defense mechanism to go repeatedly to the bathroom to make sure she hasn't wet her clothes. In this case, a complex problem involving both sex and disease, the patient did find a maladjusted solution: She escaped into chronic pain behavior.

Bill F., a successful salesman, drinks too much on a business trip to Florida and goes to bed with a prostitute. Before this, he has always been faithful to his wife. Bill, after returning home, is crucified emotionally by a deep sense of guilt that makes him impotent and miserable. His anxiety is so intolerable, it is converted into a physical pain in the groin and penis. An ill-advised surgeon thinks he has a hernia and performs a bilateral hernia repair, which leaves Bill with two painful groin scars.

By now, Bill has been given the usual prescriptions for opiates and tranquilizers, and his life is a wreck. The once-successful salesman three years later is a disabled chronic sufferer, totally impotent sexually, and totally dependent on his wife, who is now working and providing for the family. Bill F. has been emasculated by a failure to properly identify and manage the real source of his problem.

Sexuality involves a complex interplay of emotional and physical factors. It is fertile ground for excessive pain behavior to develop and flourish, unless the sufferer recognizes and overcomes the problem.

23

Common Painful Experiences: Pain and Obesity

S. L. CHAPMAN

OBESITY IS AMONG THE most severe and widespread health problems today. An estimated twenty million Americans are at least 20 percent above their ideal body-weights. These individuals face an increased risk of developing cardiovascular disease, which accounts for more than half of all deaths in the United States. Two of the leading risk factors in chronic heart disease—high blood-pressure and diabetes—often can be controlled by weight reduction alone.

Obesity is a major problem not only for heart patients but also for chronic-pain sufferers. Being overweight aggravates the problem of chronic pain in many ways. The overweight person's posture and distribution of weight put added stress on his lower-back region, which so commonly is the site of chronic pain. Many painful bone-and-joint diseases, such as osteoarthritis, are greatly improved by weight reduction, which decreases the pressure on the damaged structure and allows the afflicted person to move more easily. Overweight individuals with these kinds of disorders face an increased risk of surgery, which itself produces scarring that can cause lasting pain.

Not only does obesity aggravate the pain experience, it also hampers progress in pain-rehabilitation programs that center around physical therapy and increased activity. Overweight people find it much more difficult to do the exercises and movements necessary to make them functioning human beings again. Every movement requires more energy in an overweight person than in a normal-weight individual. This problem is especially serious in individuals with very marked obesity, who often have impaired lung-function. This can cause the blood to contain too much carbon dioxide and make such people feel constantly sleepy or lethargic.

Though not everyone who suffers from obesity or chronic pain is crippled by emotional difficulties, such problems can influence physical symptoms greatly. Excess anxiety can produce high blood-pressure, ulcers, headaches, diarrhea, and skin eruptions. Depression can lead to constipation, aches and pains, and changes in women's menstrual cycles. Emotions are closely related to a poor or good outcome for patients with physical problems. It has been found, for instance, that depressed women with cancer-like cells are more likely to develop malignant cervical cancer and die than are nondepressed women with the same cells.

The life history of an overweight person is often filled with experiences that create anxiety and depression. Jack C., who was overweight as a child, had few friends and was ridiculed by other children. Many of his teachers expected lower performance from him and gave him fewer rewards and less encouragement than they did to normal-weight children. As a consequence, Jack learned that there was little he could do to obtain satisfactions and rewards. Such a belief in one's own helplessness is a major characteristic of depressed and anxious people.

These problems are likely to persist if the person remains overweight. During adolescence, Jack had fewer dates and social activities than his peers. He was self-conscious because of his unattractive appearance and less involved in sports and other physical activities. He discovered in adulthood that he was less likely to be selected for a good job than were normal-weight persons with equal capabilities. As he gets older, he feels more intensely the physical burdens of excessive weight and faces an increased risk of chronic pain and other medical problems.

Anxiety, depression, and the low self-esteem that develop with obesity make pain more likely to occur and less likely to be treated successfully. Anxiety is common in such pain problems as tension headaches, low-back pain, and chest pain. Because anxiety is associated with muscle tension, it can play a direct role in causing and perpetuating pain problems. Many anxious people keep their muscles tense at all times and as a result they suffer from tremors, have painful movements, and tire quickly. We have previously noted this kind of circular interaction between anxiety and pain, with each one increasing the other until one is relieved. Just as anxiety and its accompanying muscular dysfunction can promote pain, the experience of pain itself causes a person to feel less in control of his life and makes him feel more anxious.

The experience of pain also is intensified by depression,

another frequent partner of obesity. Depression usually is represented by inactivity and feelings of pessimism and low self-esteem. Depressed people believe there is nothing they can do to improve their condition; they tend to remain passive and helpless. Bemoaning their woeful condition, depressed sufferers of chronic pain often stay in bed and decide that their life can only be meaningful if their pain is cured. But by staying in bed, they focus more heavily on their pain and get so accustomed to inactivity that any movement becomes painful and difficult. Thus, they do not participate actively in rehabilitation programs that demand increases in physical, social, and recreational activities: the very behaviors most likely to lift them out of their depression and focus their attention away from pain.

Guilt also can help sustain obesity and pain. Overweight individuals often are caught in a cycle of overeating and feeling guilty about overeating. Though we might expect that this guilt would lead to diminished eating, the situation is actually the reverse. The guiltier a person feels, the more he continues to overeat, almost as though he were punishing himself for overeating by forcing more food into himself.

Among chronic-pain sufferers, some view their pain as punishment that allows them to atone for past transgressions. These people often feel the most guilty and have the most pain when life is treating them well. In general, their whole lives are based on pain, humiliation, suffering, and failure.

Allowing a person to be a martyr or to atone for past sins is one of many ways in which illness can serve a useful function for someone. Staying overweight or in pain can also allow him to express anger, control other people, and avoid stress. A person can use obesity or pain subconsciously, for example, to get back at a parent who nagged him to be a social or athletic success. In some cases, illness holds marriages together. It permits an insecure spouse to feel superior to his or her sick partner and to avoid having to face his or her own inadequacies or failings.

A spouse might also encourage eating or pain behavior to make sure his or her partner stays unattractive and does not run off with someone else. A very common pattern seen with pain is one in which a whole marital relationship seems to revolve around the problem of pain. One partner plays the role of the selfless care-giver who is always there to provide comfort and support and do everything for the afflicted spouse. The other partner is always passive and always in pain and accepts gratefully the "benevolence" of the other while continuing to suffer. Similarly, in marriages with one obese partner, it is common for the nonobese spouse always to give helpful advice about what should or should not be eaten and for the obese one to listen gratefully and show token compliance but still find that he or she "just cannot seem to get this problem licked." The need to give help or to remain helpless overpowers all other needs in these marriages.

Obesity and pain can reduce stress by allowing an individual to blame failures on physical problems rather than taking direct responsibility for them. For example, a person who finds it distressing that he has few meaningful relationships in life may find it convenient to tell himself that this failure is attributable to obesity or to his need to restrict social activities because his pain may act up. Society often encourages people to escape responsibility or avoid stress by granting disability or workmen's-compensation payments to individuals in pain. Many who apply for such payments are pleased to get away from stressful, unpleasant work settings.

Unfortunately, the costs of continuing to overeat and

of showing excessive pain behavior usually exceed the benefits. A marriage in which two people play reciprocal roles of selfless care-giver and passive care-recipient is stagnant and unlikely to meet many of the couple's needs. Strong resentments are likely to build up, especially when a crisis or change in life-situation demands a more flexible behavior. Similarly, the person who avoids responsibility for his loneliness or helplessness will never find a way to become less lonely or less helpless. The person who uses pain to avoid unpleasant work is likely to feel incompetent and unproductive and to center his life more and more around pain.

A striking characteristic of overweight people and chronic-pain sufferers is the extent to which they tend to be prisoners rather than masters of their environment. In comparison with normal-weight individuals, overweight people have been found to eat less according to their physiologic hunger and more according to situations they are in or emotions they are experiencing. They eat because food is in front of them or because it is attractively displayed; they eat because they are used to eating while watching television and the television is on, or because it is a certain time of day, or because they are bored. Thus their eating is a response to their environment and not an activity under their own control.

24

Common Painful Experiences: Cancer Pain

E. E. SAMMONS

ONE OF EVERY FOUR people will contract cancer during his or her lifetime. An estimated 675,000 new cases and 351,000 deaths from this disease occurred in the United States in the most recent year for which figures are available. Mortality from cancer in adults is second only to heart disease and is larger than the combined total of the next two causes of death—stroke and accidents.

Cancer's onset is insidious, as shown by the "seven danger signals" publicized by the American Cancer Society:

1. Sore that does not heal within two weeks.
2. Change in bowel habits.
3. Lump or thickness in breast or elsewhere.
4. Unexplained bleeding or discharge from any body orifice.

5. Persistent indigestion or difficulty in swallowing.
6. Persistent hoarseness or cough for over two weeks.
7. Any change in size, color, or appearance of a wart or mole.

Pain is not a common symptom early in the disease and does not serve to warn the victim. The very name of the disease suggests a creeping, progressive, frightening process that is "crab-like." Most people know it to result in deformity, surgical mutilation, and prolonged treatment with great expense and often uncontrollable pain before a protracted death. These ideas are the basis of a national "cancer phobia" that may improve cancer awareness and early diagnosis but often provokes severe emotional storms after the diagnosis is made.

In his book *The Management of Pain,* John Bonica tells how cancer pain may develop. Direct compression or infiltration of nervous structures often produces a continuous, sharp, boring-type pain. This may be mild in the early stages and confused with arthritis or minor injury, later becoming more severe depending on the growth rate of the tumor and nervous structures involved.

A tumor metastatic to a bone (carried by blood or lymphatics from a primary site to a bone) or a cancer originating on a bone usually gives severe, continuous, dull, and deep pain of an intermittent lancinating (shooting or piercing) character. Pressure on the area or movement of the limb or spine aggravates the pain.

Obstruction of blood vessels or lymphatics is a common cause of pain in cancer cases. Blockage of an artery gives a numbness, weakness, and deep-aching discomfort secondary to decreased blood supply and inadequate oxygenation to the area involved. Motion of the affected body part tends to aggravate the misery. Venous or lymphatic obstruction causes swelling, engorgement, tightness, and fullness of the body part, with a bluish-red or plethoric appearance.

A particular type of pain is produced when a cancer mass obstructs a portion of the intestinal tract. Dilation of the proximal (nearer the stomach) portion of the bowel causes distention of the abdomen and gripping, variable, and continuous pain. Nausea and weakness are prominent as the process worsens.

Swelling and thickening in areas containing many pain-sensitive structures, such as fascia (connective tissues) or periosteum (bone-covering tissue), is an important mechanism of pain production with cancer.

The neck is an example of a part of the body susceptible to such pain. Blood vessels and nerves inside the head are another. Dull, aching, progressive pain is characteristic.

Tumors in some body areas may occasionally cause excruciating pain by leading to necrosis (localized death) of tissues, infection, and inflammation. Oral, vaginal, and rectal structures are common examples; also the ear or eye.

Perhaps most frequently associated with pain are bone tumors, either primary or metastatic. An expanding lesion irritating and stretching the nerve-rich periosteum gives a constant, aching, deep sensation difficult to tolerate. Osteosarcoma, which produces this type of pain, is a rapidly growing cancer originating in the bone. Breast and prostate cancer can metastasize to the vertebrae, to the bones of the extremities, or to the pain-sensitive portions of the brain and skull. Melanoma (cancer of a pigmented mole) may also put rapidly growing lesions in all of these structures. Tumors of the kidney occasionally spread to the bone.

Other examples are: (1) stomach cancer—burning, ulcer-type pain; (2) pancreas—a vague aching in the upper-back region and pit of stomach, with feelings of indigestion, excess stomach acidity, and burning; (3) intestinal tumor—may obstruct bowel, with griping pain and bloating; (4) lung cancer—often involves the sensitive covering of the lungs (pleura) or the bones of the rib cage, also may occlude air passages and blood vessels leading to pneumonia and resultant pleural irritation; (5) bladders—fullness, burning, and irritation; (6) uterus or uterine cervix (neck of womb)—pelvic pressure and bladder irritation in late states.

Cancers not frequently associated with pain are those of the larynx, esophagus, liver, lymphatic tissues, blood-forming tissues, muscles, and reproductive organs.

Therapy for relief of cancer pain is usually directed into three areas:

1. Adequate systemic drug therapy is often necessary to relieve the debilitating limitations caused by the disease while maintaining a minimum of drug side-effects. Undesirable effects are produced mostly by the opiates and include drowsiness, lethargy, loss of interest in normally pleasant daily activities, decreased sexual interest, loss of appetite, weight loss, and constipation. When an opiate is needed, methadone is probably a drug of choice because of its longer-lasting effects, which cover the patient's analgesic needs more completely around the clock. Aspirin and acetaminophen can often give acceptable pain relief without the problems of the opiates. Phenothiazine drugs such as Mellaril may be helpful to control severe states of agitated depression. Nerve blocks can supplement or replace drug therapy; one advantage is their complete absence of narcotizing side-effects.
2. Surgical procedures may result in removal or

containment of the disease, relieve dysfunction (such as an intestinal obstruction), or provide debridement of an infected, necrotic area of the body invaded by a tumor. Special neurosurgical procedures for pain relief, such as chordotomy and rhizotomy, should be limited to the late stages of the metastatic disease.

3. Radiation therapy and chemotherapy may temporarily stop a cancer growth or reduce its size. In recent years there has been a vigorous attack on cancer by medical science and many supporting groups that has resulted in earlier diagnosis, better surgical treatment, new forms of drug therapy, and improved radiation therapy. One in four cancer patients were cured twenty-five years ago, but now the figure is one in three, equaling a saving of 55,000 lives per year. New specialists, known as oncologists, with a background in internal medicine coordinate the medical treatment of cancer. More people are surviving the disease for longer periods, so in this sense the attack is successful.

But what of the quality of life remaining to the cancer victim? How is he to deal with his disease and its effects on his daily life, work, family, and every other facet of his existence? It is important to keep in mind that the cancer victim is still a whole person and must be treated as such. Simply attacking the disease often overlooks this concept. Rehabilitation toward normal or near-normal life functions should be the common target of patient, family, and physician. The overall plan of pain relief will depend greatly on the attitude of the patient toward his disease and on his desire to return to more functional, meaningful living.

Analogy to the pain of childbirth comes to mind. The

childbirth experience varies along the whole spectrum from acceptance and tolerance of pain to feelings of unbearable suffering. The cancer victim may come to accept his pain and derive great personal satisfaction from bearing it with courage and fortitude, or he may demand all the physician has to offer, plus more.

In any case, the patient must be thoroughly informed as to the potential good and bad effects of every form of therapy proposed. He should understand the procedure as completely as possible and participate in decisions regarding its use and timing. This enhances greatly his emotional well-being and the total value of the therapy.

One of the most common mistakes in handling cancer sufferers is to instruct them to cut back their daily activities and remain in bed as long as they wish. Prolonged bed rest *per se* is often conducive to various malfunctions of vital organs, such as increased risk of lung and blood-clotting defects. Rest in bed is frequently made necessary by early drug abuse but not justified by the actual disease growth.

A program of daily activities will keep the cancer patient out of bed and engaged in pleasurable actions as much as possible. Such a program can be very important in relieving the emotional agony of the patient and so actually decrease his feelings of pain.

Fear and a sense of helplessness often keep the patient from planning and participating in things he is perfectly able to do and would enjoy doing. Simple counseling will often persuade the patient to take a hike or auto trip, or attend entertaining, social, or religious events that he may otherwise think are inadvisable. Proper activities may afford pleasure to him and to his family members and increase his feeling of well-being. Opportunities to meet and talk with loved ones may relieve some of his interpersonal worries and give him a chance to settle some of his nagging affairs. Meaningful at-home reading or hobbies may diminish drug needs and make circumstances much more easy and pleasant. Certain exercises or relaxation techniques to promote tranquility and sleep can be valuable.

Following the lead of England and European countries, there is currently a rapidly growing interest in the United States in providing a new type of care for the patient with cancer, for whom further medical or surgical treatment is inappropriate. This concept of care has perhaps been best integrated under the term "hospice," meaning a way station for the traveler. The focus is upon humanitarian concern for the patient and his family and incorporates ethical considerations of respect for the individual, inclusion in a loving community, concern for bodily needs, and considerations of a higher and broader purpose of life. Home care by visiting nurses, readily available in-patient care, inclusion of the family as the primary care unit, pain control, and attention to spiritual needs are some of the uppermost considerations in the hospice concept of patient care. This means of lovingly helping the patient to cope with what Kübler-Ross calls the "final stage of personal growth" is a program of tremendous potential human value.

To illustrate how different people endure incurable cancer in different ways, the following case histories, all of them actual but given fictitious names, are presented.

Will S., a fifty-year-old white male veteran of World War II, noticed a small, painless mass in the tissues below his right jaw. For a few weeks he did nothing except see a general practitioner, who give him a salve to apply locally.

As the size of the lesion increased, he consulted a physician at a large medical center and a diagnosis of cancer of the neck was made.

Radical neck dissection followed by radiation therapy was recommended and carried out by careful surgeons who conveyed a sense of good care and thoroughness to the patient. Will responded well and was back on his feet. After almost ten years of cautious optimism, it was decided that for all practical purposes he was "cured."

When hoarseness and trouble in swallowing then appeared, Will, now sixty, was devastated when a removal of his larynx was recommended. Losing his voice, adjusting to a tracheostomy, professional disability, and perhaps worst of all, the prospect of the return of the initial disease process, all combined to overwhelm him. He was reduced to a state of hopelessness and depression from which he never really recovered. His sense of self-worth and his value as a civic leader and field representative of a large automobile-manufacturing company were virtually destroyed. A strong basic religious faith and loving support from his small family were important positive factors at this point in Will's life.

With appearance of a lung metastasis three years later and a shift to the surgical care of a physician who spent little time with the personal needs of his patient, Will's helplessness and depression deepened. Verbal communication became unbearably awkward. His lung was removed; this had many negative and probably no positive effects. The restriction of a quick and active mind to communication by writing or sign language had been frustrating to the patient for the last three years, and now his new problems reduced Will to an emasculated, mutilated shadow of his former self. He displayed anger and rage frequently, directed mostly at his circumstances in general.

Physical pain was never a prominent part of Will's disease. Analgesics and sleep medication for his surgical pain were all he seemed to require or want. His emotional pain was extreme, however. At some point, probably just before his laryngectomy, the significance to Will of the future loss of his voice was put aside or ignored in the effort to attack the disease. He never had time or opportunity to discuss, consider, and participate in major decisions regarding further therapy. His later strong resentment over the mutilation of his vocal cords was apparent to everyone.

With proper, thoughtful consideration, Will could easily have decided to dispense with further expensive, time-consuming, physically and emotionally mutilating treatment and turned to face death as a dignified human being, probably even with personal heroism. Doctors do not always consider the whole patient, and patients too often trust their doctors too much. With proper care, Will might have been helped to avoid the extreme emotional pain, suffering, and torture he finally endured. He died in a matter of hours after onset of acute respiratory failure.

Mrs. Sue K., a fifty-four-year-old widowed mother of two adult sons, went to her local general practitioner complaining of a feeling of ill health. Mild anemia was found and treated with iron, without success. A second evaluation revealed a lung shadow and referral was made to a thoracic surgeon. Diagnosis of an inoperable bronchogenic cancer (arising from an air tube) was made. There was a recommendation of chemotherapy (anticancer drugs), to be started when Mrs. K. was hospitalized within a few days.

The diagnosis was met by considerable shock and disbelief on the part of the patient. She expressed the feeling that she had always been a good Christian, never smoked, and did not see why this had to happen to her. She asked angrily why the initial check-up had not revealed the cancer. Grief and depression were evident in her prolonged crying and sobbing for a period of days. This continued until she recovered from the nausea and weakness brought on by chemotherapy.

Soon afterward, Mrs. K. suddenly sat up straight, appeared calm, smiled strongly, and declared that this was God's will for her and she would accept it. She wrote a short but clear will including all those people, near or far, whom she loved. She sought and welcomed counsel from ministers who had had a part in her life. She gave a concise, handwritten booklet to each of her sons, to be opened after her death, saying a final goodbye and expressing wishes about personal matters not covered in her will. When all this was done, she relaxed, read mostly religious literature, visited friends, and generally enjoyed the courageous attitude toward death she had assumed.

Mrs. K. did not again complain of pain or discomfort, although fluid was drained from her chest cavities on two occasions and the chemotherapy regimen was repeated once. She died of pneumonia after six months of stabilized health. Undoubtedly, her minimal medical and surgical intervention and strong support from family, ministers, and friends, plus her own courageous faith in ultimate good were decisive in her confrontation of impending death.

Jim C., a twenty-one-year-old Caucasian male high-school graduate, living with his parents and engaged to be married, complained of a painless mass on the left side of his neck. Biopsy of the neck lesion proved to be teratocarcinoma originating in the testicle, a particularly malignant tumor that invades tissues locally and metastasizes to distant body parts. Radiation therapy was first performed, then surgery for radical neck dissection was done.

A period of remission from disease followed. Seven months after the original biopsy a large mass was discovered in a space near Jim's kidneys. Excision and examination of this tumor revealed it to be the same-type cancer as the original. Treatment with chemotherapeutic agents produced a second disease-remission.

Eleven months after this episode Jim began to complain of left-flank pain, despite no objective evidence of disease recurrence. The pain was described as sharp, superficial, and steady, being worse in the evenings and interfering with sleep. It was eased by a heating pad, "deep heat" rub, and by Percodan, an oral narcotic drug that the patient began taking five or six times a day. His appetite decreased, loss of weight was apparent, and Jim was depressed, partially because of his hopeless, recurring physical problems and partially as an inevitable side-effect of the narcotic drug. He ended his vigorous pursuit of leisure activities and tended to remain in bed for all but two hours a day.

When examined in the Emory University Pain Control Center, he appeared depressed and assumed a slumped posture. His abdomen was difficult to examine because of "guarding," a reflex that tightens the abdominal muscles when the peritoneum, or lining of the inner abdominal wall, is inflamed. No abdominal mass could be detected.

Narcotic withdrawal was prescribed, to be followed by a series of nerve blocks and supportive care for pain relief and a hopeful return to a more active life with less depression. Hospitalization for Percodan withdrawal was thought advisable, but after a discussion of this the patient decided to withdraw at home. A full twelve days was recommended, dropping one Percodan tablet each day. In case of difficulty he was to call the clinic for help. To everyone's surprise, Jim withdrew from all drugs in only four days, and returned to the clinic two days after that. His father reported that Jim had just climbed Stone Mountain with his fiancée (the trail up the mountain is approximately one and one-half miles long) and was feeling remarkably better.

Indeed, Jim's general health indicators (increased activities, decreased drug use, decreased pain complaints, and increased optimism) were much improved. His pain experience had not worsened. Over a ten-day period, he received four nerve blocks, one a placebo, which gave him considerable relief. He estimated a 70 percent improvement after the series of blocks and was down to only four aspirin tablets a day. He remained improved functionally, was asked to call the pain clinic should his pain experience worsen, and was cautioned to avoid narcotics. A supportive block every two weeks was scheduled.

About one month later, an intestinal obstruction requiring surgical relief occurred. Incisional pain and right abdominal pain was severe. Methadone provided adequate pain relief with minimal "drugging" or "narcotizing" effects and could, as soon as the healing process after surgery permitted, be administered orally.

Jim presented himself for no further nerve blocks and continued taking methadone, reporting by phone that he was still in satisfactory condition. In another five months, Jim had his final illness, followed shortly by death. The entire process of disease and death had taken twenty-seven months.

The most significant achievements in this young man's illness seemed to be his ability to overcome his "death-like" state of narcotic overusage and his resumption of active life, brief as it was. He withdrew from drugs, felt better, and made the most of his last months with a decision to live each day for itself. He displayed no sense of defeat and no morbid attitude.

To elaborate on the emotional storm associated with cancer, the feelings of a person who contracts cancer can be better understood by observing an individual in the process of dying as outlined by Dr. Elisabeth Kübler-Ross. Indeed, the cancer patient either is beginning the accelerated process of dying or believes that he is doing so, based on the common and widespread fear of this disease.

On discovering in himself one of the seven danger signals of cancer, the first reaction of Tom J. is to deny his discovery by saying, in effect, "Oh, this couldn't be anything serious. I'm sure it will be all right." This denial may continue for some time, until his symptoms are definitely worse or until a third party uses his influence on the patient to seek medical evaluation. Initial evaluation by a doctor may be inconclusive and the mental mechanism of denial continues operating to protect Tom from severe anxiety.

As the disease progresses so that doubts pick away at his constant denying and ignoring of what is taking place, Tom is examined again. This time a specific test or biopsy indicates cancer of a rapidly malignant form. The response is anger. "Oh, no! Why me? What have I done to deserve this? I have too much to do to be sick!" All these thoughts and feelings are typical expressions of the anger and rage building up in the patient. Tom's denial in itself is a confirmation that he actually has a deadly disease. Surgery offers some hope statistically, and he accepts and plans for an operation, perhaps jumping back and forth between denial and anger as he awaits and then experiences initial surgery. The message may then be from the surgeon, "I think we got it all. Things look good." Relief replaces fear and optimism grows.

Tom, however, continues to vacillate between tormenting feelings of denial, fear, and anger, sometimes deciding that everything is going to be all right and sometimes feeling doomed, helpless, hopeless. Of course, his family, friends, and physician experience all these feelings as well—in varying degrees. Their counsel, comments, relating of personal experiences, and efforts to cheer up the victim all have helpful effects on Tom's feelings.

The patient is now assessing himself frequently for new findings and evidence of the disease, and begins the third emotional phase, that of bargaining. "God, if you will let me be cured, I will be a new person, go to church every Sunday, spend more time with my children, contribute large sums to the Cancer Society, mend my dishonest ways," and so forth. Tom now is more and more accepting that he has a fatal illness but is hoping for a "miracle" to get out of it. Pleading, fearful, begging prayers are offered. He may bargain openly or surreptitiously with his surgeon, the message taking the form of "check me carefully, operate your best, get rid of this disease for me and I will (*a*) pay whatever you ask, (*b*) be eternally grateful, (*c*) praise you highly to others," and the like. He is, in short, not certain whether he is doomed or has a chance for cure, and is still trying to escape.

A persistent question, not yet answered to everyone's satisfaction, is whether Tom should be told that he is dying. That this should even be a question is hard to understand from the point of view of facing honestly and squarely all of life's trials and realities. Perhaps the question is asked improperly and should really be, "When and how do we openly discuss death and dying with the patient?" We are all dying from the moment we are born, but at different rates and with different degrees of perception and awareness of the process.

At some point in the cancer process, the patient will know he is dying and even have a fairly good idea of how fast without being told. Just as it would be undesirable to remove hope from a patient when chances of help or even cure are present (regardless of how remote), it would also be cruel, confusing, and thoughtless not to assist the patient in understanding the likely outcome as indicated by available evidence. The physician serves a dubious and probably deceitful purpose if he misleads the patient and family and gives them false hopes. He simply keeps the patient from entering and experiencing the final emotional processes of death and dying—those that may lead to the most meaningful changes in the patient's life. The only possible gain from false hope is avoiding the issue of death, and this is, of course, a loss of opportunity for the patient to begin to prepare himself.

Later there are more symptoms and signs of Tom's disease, such as weight loss and progressive malaise (feeling of ill health). After consultation with his doctor, evidence becomes unmistakable that the malignancy is still present and metastasizing or spreading to distant body sites. Surgery has brought varying degrees of mutilation, loss of body functions, pain, and great expense. Tom now enters the fourth emotional stage—depression. His frustration is overwhelming. He knows he is going to die and will probably do so soon. Minor painful perceptions are converted to major pain-complaints.

He cries, wrings his hands, and grieves for his lost life and hopes that will never be realized. He may see his family and friends experience similar depression and grief. Regrettably, they may begin too early to separate themselves from him. This emotional separation deepens the patient's feelings of hopelessness, helplessness, loneliness, and depression. The family has perhaps begun to do what the patient may do next, depending on his background and personality, and that is to accept his disease and the fact that he is about to die.

This is the point at which the attitudes of the victim, physician, and family make all the difference. Dr. Kübler-Ross cites evidence and experience that dying patients may display sudden new radiance, vigor, and cheerfulness. Pain complaints diminish. This is not simple resignation to disease and surrender to death, but acceptance that death is coming and it is all right. A change has taken place to the extent that the person knows what is happening is natural and therefore right, and need not be feared.

As apprehension subsides, positive outlooks can now predominate, and it is possible that the person will undergo many changes of attitudes, reconcile past errors or grievances, and in general begin a healthy preparation for his impending death. Financial affairs may be put in order, a will carefully made, discussions with the family held, and funeral preferences stated. The dying person may even be glad that his crisis—this "dark night of the soul"—has led him to this point. He may become an example to all of how to die with dignity and courage. There may be feelings of peace, satisfaction, and victory at facing and overcoming this ultimate test, this "final stage of learning" in life.

25

Lessons from the Great Religions

S. F. BRENA

ELSEWHERE IN THIS BOOK the concept of self-esteem has been mentioned in its relation to chronic states of anxiety and depression. We've pointed out that low self-esteem may be at the root of various maladjusted behaviors, such as obesity, sexual inadequacy, and chronic pain. Anxiety and depression have been discussed from behavioral and psychoanalytic points of view. In this chapter, we will talk about these concepts in the framework of the great religions.

In building our self-esteem, we go through various stages of maturation. The newborn child is not aware of himself as a separate entity; all he wants is to have his needs met without giving anything in exchange. This stage of development is sometimes called "animal awareness." In late childhood and early adolescence, the child learns to know himself as a separate being with a body different from all other bodies; he also learns to be "lovable," that is, to give something—a smile, small services—in return for the gratification of his needs and desires. Despite his being "lovable," he is basically self-centered and expects all things he receives from the outside to add to his well-being.

At the onset of mature adulthood, he learns to integrate his feelings with the use of reason, based on ethical and moral codes rather than selfish wants and desires. This is the stage of "moral-awareness." It is followed by a higher stage of "love-awareness," in which the individual learns to interact with other people, not only on the level of morality, but mainly in terms of love expressed through unselfish service.

Love-awareness, however, is more than humanitarian service: It is an actual realization of our true spiritual nature. We come to know ourselves not only as a body but also as a soul, thus we are able to recognize other people as distinct souls who share our spiritual identity. The difference between simple "humanitarian" love and love-awareness may be difficult to grasp and can be demonstrated as follows: If we engage in humanitarian service only to gratify ourselves, to "feel good," and expect praise and rewards from those who receive our help, we are acting from a lower stage of maturity. We may be "lovable" but remain childish. On the other hand, if we serve others in a spirit of detachment, doing so because they are fellow human beings, we operate from a state of true love-awareness. The distinction is not merely academic—it is crucial in our understanding of the inner meaning of all spiritual teachings.

The ultimate meaning of love is the realization of

equality among men and unity in creation. As a biological function, love is energy, a dynamic force binding all creation together, an essential part of life. In the human society, love-consciousness is first expressed in family life, then within a community, up toward a national identity, until it finally reaches a universal, cosmic awareness.

We can think of the building of self-esteem essentially as an ascent of morality and an emergence of love; a movement from self-centered, narcissistic attitudes toward more unselfish, love-motivated expressions. It is an unending life process in which we learn to deal with others not in terms of our desires or real or imagined needs, but in terms of moral choices based on ethical codes. All religions stress this process as having the deepest religious significance; it is the cornerstone of a truly integrated, honest, spiritual life.

The Ten Commandments and the Sermon on the Mount provide moral guidance and a call to love-awareness in the Judeo-Christian civilization. They find their equivalent, almost to the word, in the rules of Yama and Niyama—forbearance, not-killing, veracity, not-stealing, continence, not-coveting (Yama); and purification, contentment, austerity, devotion, and unselfish service (Niyama). These points are made in the Yoga Sutra of Patanjali, one of the holy books of Hinduism.

Failure to grow in adulthood—failure to function morally in a relationship of love with our fellow men—causes defects in our personal self-esteem. It makes our self-esteem more likely to break down in the face of challenge. Two examples can be used here.

If we engage in humanitarian service with a desire for payoff—prestige and high standing in our church community, for instance—but fail to get a reward, we feel frustrated, anxious about what went wrong in our scheming, and eventually depressed because our desires have not been fulfilled. Somatization and conversion of our maladjusted feelings into physical symptoms are then likely, laying the ground for pain and suffering.

On the other hand, if we perform service to others from a mental attitude of silent love and immediately forget about it, nothing can hurt us, because love-energy and not the wish for payoff has motivated our action.

Slowly and almost reluctantly, medical science has started to recognize the impact of love-energy—or rather the lack of it—on our health. In his well-documented book *The Broken Heart,* James J. Lynch presents evidence of a relationship between marital status and death rates from various diseases. Lonely people are more prone to develop coronary-artery disease, cerebrovascular disease, and hypertension. Death rates for almost every type of cancer are significantly higher in lonely individuals, according to Lynch, who bases his statements on 1960 U.S. population data.

Other information drawn from studies by the National Program to Conquer Heart Disease, Cancer, and Stroke shows that the state of Nevada, which has the second-highest level of education and median level of income (for the age range 25–64), has the highest death rate in the country for white males and females (1960 census), while the neighboring state of Utah, with similar environmental conditions, has one of the lowest death rates in the United States. In his book *Who Shall Live?,* Victor Fuchs has pointed out that Utah has a relatively stable standard of living, rooted in deep religious feelings. It is a state where family ties are strong and marriages are generally secure; on the other hand, Nevada is one of the divorce centers of America, with 20 percent of the male population, ages 35–64, living lonely lives.

In current psychoanalytic thought, states of anxiety and depression are related to the so-called guilt-complex, which is recognized as a root cause of these kinds of maladaptive emotional syndromes. In his book *Clinical Psychiatry and Religion,* E. M. Pattison defines various types of guilt. Psychological guilt is a feeling of condemnation by one's own conscience; existential guilt is a state of denial of one's social nature; ontological guilt is a maladaptive recognition of one's own imperfection. But the doctrine of the guilt-complex as the root of most neurotic, painful, psychosomatic illnesses stands at cross-purposes with teachings of the Holy Scriptures, which indicate that in the consciousness of sin lies the basis of evil. God does not punish us for our imperfection; we punish ourselves in our refusal to live up to our wholesome human potential as members of a universal society of living creatures.

The scriptures of all spiritual religions provide commandments, models, guidelines, sermons, parables, and discourses that are strikingly similar in tracing the path of enlightenment toward a balanced life of inner peace, productivity, and joy. All the great religions agree, even if they use different symbols to express the same truth, that we are a soul manifested through the working of the mind in the vehicle of the body. These religions also affirm that most men live unaware of their true spiritual nature. Because they are so grossly immersed in their body-consciousness, they are totally ignorant of their soul-consciousness. In this ignorance, the roots of all pain and suffering lie. All religions teach a spiritual training to help man retrace his way to his true divine nature, the soul; in doing so, he will eradicate forever the source of all sorrows.

In an earlier chapter of this book, on the anatomy of pain, the role of intelligent brain activity in controlling feelings and emotional forces was mentioned. Failure of the neocortex to govern the visceral brain was viewed as an important source of malfunction. These statements do not mean that intelligent behavior always brings health, prosperity, and happiness. If this were true, super-intelligent people should have enjoyed a pain-free, well-adjusted life. A survey of history shows that, more often than not, the lives of philosophers, artists, and men of genius were filled with self-created miseries. For example, Friedrich Nietzsche (1844–1900), the philosopher of the "superman," with his theories of intellectual excellence, died insane after years of great loneliness, inner struggle, and suffering. The intellect is like a double-edged blade: It can badly hurt those who use it carelessly.

Again, the lives of famous people reveal that those able to match intelligent creative activity with wisdom and submission to their deity did show evidence of inner peace and a balanced personality; this can be inferred from their writings and from the patterns of their lives.

The Founding Fathers of the United States, in their Declaration of Independence, relied on "the protection of the Divine Providence" when they mutually pledged to each other their "lives, fortunes, and sacred honor." The republic they founded and placed "under God" has lasted two hundred years and is now one of the mightiest on earth. A few years after the American Revolution, the French people led their own revolution in the name of the same human rights, chopped off their king's head, banned God, and placed their newly founded French Republic under the guidance of Reason. That republic lasted less than ten years and ended in bloody madness of the Terror and the Napoleonic Wars.

Obviously, there must be another dimension in the makeup of the human entity: one not found under the knife of anatomist or surgeon, one that cannot be analyzed in the laboratory, one that can only be felt and experienced inwardly. It is something that lights up the path of intelligent activity and guides human beings through the challenges of life. The testimony of saints and sages of all religions indicates this inner, sacred source of wisdom to be the soul.

One of the holy books that stands out as a masterpiece of wisdom and practical values is the Bhagavad-Gita, the Hindu gospel that is closest to the Judeo-Christian tradition. The Gita is a discourse on the art of right living and right thinking between Arjuna, prince of India, and Lord Krishna, the Christ-like deity of the Hindu. Historically, the Bhagavad-Gita is part of a religious drama called Mahabharata, one of the poetic literary masterpieces that have exalted mankind on a few occasions. In the Gita, spiritual ascent is viewed as an individual effort in a personal relationship with God through right work, devotional love, and the development of wisdom by prayer and meditation.

Right work is defined as work done for service and not for gain only, with a mental attitude of inner renunciation in which the fruits of labor are not considered a personal property but a gift from God. The Old Testament has the same statement about the mystique of work, as we can read in Ecclesiastes 2:24: "There is nothing better for a man. . . . that he should make his soul enjoy good in his labour. This also I saw, that it was from the hand of God."

In the concept of worship through work, we find an agreement with contemporary psychology, which views work-pride—work done well for the joy of it, not for greed—as an important cornerstone in the building of a mature personality. All the great religions have acknowledged the role of work in maintaining a balanced personality, open to moral and spiritual calls. St. Paul put it strongly in his second letter to the Thessalonians: "This we commanded you, that if any would not work, neither should he eat . . . and exhort by our Lord Jesus Christ, that with quietness they work, and eat their own bread."

In an ill-advised compassionate trend, Western society today has gone too far in passing laws granting monetary compensation for escape from work via pain complaints in excess of objective, demonstrable disease. Years ago, at the Emory Pain Control Center, we began to see the wisdom of St. Paul's instructions to work for a living. We started documenting the devastating effects of learned sick-behaviors and related feelings of worthlessness on potentially able workers who were trapped in a nightmare of welfare lifestyles.

Devotional love is another important step on the path to spiritual enlightenment, stressed in both the Bhagavad-Gita and the Old and New Testaments. The seventh chapter of the Gita dwells mainly on the process of knowledge of the Absolute through devotion, and the twelfth chapter deals with devotional service as a form of active prayer. Meanwhile, the books of Psalms and the Song of Solomon in the Old Testament echo the Gita's chapters on devotional love almost to the letter. But nowhere in all the holy scriptures can a discourse on devotional love be found any greater than the New Testament's Sermon on the Mount in both Matthew and Luke.

What is devotional love? Basically, it is an inner attitude of trust, faith, and surrender to an Authority greater than any human authority, a Spirit that has spoken to mankind from the beginning of time through the voices of sages and saints in all the world's cultures. From the

Chinese Book of Tao to the Muslim Koran and Jewish Talmud, from the Hindu Upanishads to the Book of Revelation, from the writings of Plotinus to those of Saint Bernard, Meister Eckart, William Blake, and thousands of others who "walked with God," the testimony is this: To achieve inner peace and joyful life, we must surrender our little selves, our selfish pretense of being at the center of the world, and start climbing the mountain of universal love. There we will come to know ourselves, not as pain-prone bodies, but as free souls untouched by sorrow and suffering. If we could truly live up to the meaning of the famous Twenty-third Psalm, rather than merely repeat it occasionally in Sunday worship services, all our destructive feelings of worthlessness, fear, anxiety, and the like would melt away.

The process of inner surrender is well-illustrated in the Book of Job. Job is an honest, law-abiding man who is devastated by a series of disasters and illnesses; he cannot easily accept them, as they appear to defy his concept of God's justice and mercy. He repeatedly tries to rationalize his hurt feelings and lamentations with several friends who bring him consolation. Finally, God speaks to Job: "Who is this that darkeneth counsel by words without knowledge? . . . Where wast thou when I laid the foundations of the earth? Declare, if thou hast understanding." The reply of Job is complete surrender: "I know that Thou canst do everything, and that no thought can be withholden from Thee. . . . Wherefore I abhor myself and repent in dust and in ashes."

People who are not informed may think inner surrender is basically a dull attitude of apathy and mental laziness. On the contrary, the active practice of morality in love-awareness gives rise to the keenest intelligence, capable of enormous, almost effortless productivity. Because we are intelligent human beings, we must exercise reason to plan our activities so that they will result in the best service to us and to others, since we share with mankind the responsibility to think and act. As we think, plan, work, or play, our mental attitude should always be one of detachment. It should be as though we were simultaneously the actors on the stage and the spectators in the orchestra seats, able to have an occasional good laugh at the play. Both the gospels and the Gita stress this attitude of inner detachment from our outer activities as the key point to peaceful, healthy, anxiety-free living.

Unselfish work and devotional love cannot be achieved by sheer will power and reason alone. In the unfolding of our spiritual identity, a third element is needed: prayer; in particular, that silent prayer of the heart known as meditation. Spiritual meditation is both a scientific technique and an intimate process of soul-awakening. Modern science has submitted transcendental meditation and other meditational techniques to the test of unbiased research and found that many of the ancient claims of Yoga and Zen are true. Indeed, meditation does bring remarkable changes in the activity of the sympathetic nervous system. The quieting of this system in a state of wakeful rest and relaxation can be viewed as a guidepost to better health. We must remember that an animal-like, sympathetic overreaction in a "fight or flight" type of situation has lost its survival meaning in humans today. It is now a maladaptive emotional expression, which may be harmful to health.

In prayer-meditation, a state of sharpened consciousness in a relaxed body is used to focus attention on a single idea of spiritual significance, coupled with suppression of all other thinking activity. The intensity of attention on the chosen thought should be so strong that the person meditating gradually becomes one with that thought. Some of the best-known examples of such power of meditation are offered by well-documented cases of saints. Some were able to focus their meditative attention so strongly on the wounds of the crucified Christ that they were actually able to share His suffering and mystically enjoy His love.

Regular habits of daily meditation coupled with right-thinking and service work have the subtle power, witnessed by all who have made the effort, to bring us to a unified, integrated way of life. It is one in which wisdom comes to balance our relationship with the world and guides us in making decisions. In the language of psychoanalysis, it is described as a progressive fading away of our habitual sense of identity and an expanding of consciousness into a more joyful dimension. Our ego defenses are given up as we move from a position of egocentricity into a new relationship with God and our fellow men. Reality is now seen as it is, outside the boundaries of the narcissistic ego.

The problem is that efforts in meditation must be steady and regular; our whole heart and mind must be fixed on our central idea if we wish to experience its splendid, soul-expanding effects. Here again, one of the paradoxes of our human nature is evident: We want health but we rarely honestly commit ourselves to a life-style conducive to this desired state of health. We want to experience peace, joy, and prosperity, but shy away when told what we must do to achieve spiritual growth: that unique way that nobody can travel for us, a way that each must go in his own intimate personal path.

Comparative studies of both Eastern and Western religions show that all religions agree on the view that human health is mainly a function of the individual's commitment to a lifestyle governed by self-control and wisdom rather than by unchecked, negative feelings and related emotional storms. Our self-esteem is not a static structure in which states of personal growth are fixed steps never to be retraced again. Our growth is an evolutionary process; it continues throughout our lives. We usually commute back and forth between selfishness and more mature expressions of love-awareness, but the more our personality is rooted in a spiritual commitment, the less wide and disturbing is the swing.

Human life is an up-and-down experience in which we find ourselves in a deep and dark ravine one day and on top of the mountain the next, with a glorious view all around. Pain can be a positive experience, warning us that something is wrong not only in our body but also in our whole way of living. If we interpret the signals constructively, we can quickly leave our downward path and go on to an upward journey. The price we pay for failure to rise from decline is chronic pain and grief.

Our nervous system is the common channel through which both grief and joy are felt. The "spinal-gate" theory tells us we can govern our sensory input and screen out overloads if we properly use our brain; perceptual experiences can thus be either converted into regressive, maladaptive behaviors or result in love-oriented, integrated behaviors of spiritual significance.

In all of us, no matter how mature we've grown, there are "breaking points." We can only take "so much," and after that we are bound to fall into a pit of anxiety-depression, where chronic pain becomes our crutch. Regular habits of meditation and unselfish work can strengthen us against the harmful influences of stress.

The lives of the world's saints and sages show many episodes of fortitude in which each crisis was followed by a quick surge toward higher states of consciousness, not through "fight-or-flight" responses, but through acceptance and spiritual surrender. Jesus came close to His own breaking point when he was standing in Gethsemane and "began to be sorrowful and very heavy."

St. Luke, a physician, has given us a vivid picture of Jesus' crisis, describing the symptoms of His acute anxiety-state on the Mount of Olives: "And being in agony, he prayed more earnestly: and his sweat was as it were great drops of blood falling down to the ground." At this point Jesus is close to asking for escape: "O my Father, if it be possible, let this cup pass from me, nevertheless not as I will, but as Thou wilt." He looks around for support from his friends and disciples, but finds them asleep. Jesus acknowledges how vain it is to rely on outer sources of strength: "The spirit indeed is willing, but the flesh is weak."

Jesus prayed again, saying: "O my Father, if this cup may not pass away from me, except I drink it, Thy will be done." The crisis is over, the agony is gone, the acceptance of impending suffering and death is unconditional. Peace is restored to His heart so that He can now quietly wake up the disciples: "Rise, let us be going: behold, he is at hand that doth betray me." In accepting the Cross, Jesus sets the stage for the glory of the Resurrection, and leaves a perfect model for the acceptance of pain without emotional distress for all centuries to come.

References

CHAPTER 1

Bonica, J. J. Introduction to *Advances in Neurology*, vol. 4. New York: Raven Press, 1974.
Brena, S. F. "Pain: What's New?" *Southern Medicine*, October 1975, pp. 27–33.
Hirsch, T. "The Billion Dollar Backache." *National Safety News*, May 1977, pp. 51–54.
———. *Work in America*. Report of a Special Task Force to the Secretary of Health, Education and Welfare. Cambridge, Mass.: M.I.T. Press, 1973.

CHAPTER 2

Bois, J. S. *The Art of Awareness*. Dubuque: W. C. Brown, 1973.
———. *Breeds of Men: Toward the Adulthood of Humankind*. New York: Harper & Row, 1970.

Chase, S. and M. T. Chase. *Power of Words.* New York: Harcourt, Brace and World, 1954.

CHAPTER 3

Brena, S. F.; W. Hammonds; I. P. Unikel, "Compensation for Work-related Injuries and the Rehabilitation of Patients with Chronic Pain." *Southern Medical Journal.*

Fordyce, W. *Behavioral Methods for Control of Chronic Pain and Illness.* St. Louis: C. V. Mosby, 1976.

Melzack, R. *The Puzzle of Pain: Revolution in Theory and Treatment.* New York: Basic Books, 1973.

Miller, N. E. "Learning of Visceral and Glandular Responses." *Science* 163 (1969), pp. 434–45.

CHAPTER 4

Bowers, K. S. "Pain, Anxiety and Perceived Control." *Journal of Consulting and Clinical Psychology* 32 (1968), pp. 596–602.

Seligman, M. E. P. *Helplessness: On Depression, Development and Death.* San Francisco: W. H. Freeman & Co., 1975.

Sternbach, R. A. *Pain Patients: Traits and Treatments.* New York: Academic Press, 1974.

CHAPTER 5

Beecher, H. A. "Pain: One Mystery Solved." *Science* 151 (1966), pp. 840–41.

Frank, J. D. *Persuasion and Healing: A Comparative Study of Psychotherapy.* 2nd rev. ed. Baltimore: Johns Hopkins Press, 1973.

Halpern, L. M. "Psychotropic Drugs and the Management of Chronic Pain." In *Advances in Neurology,* vol. 4. New York: Raven Press, 1974.

Jarvis, D. C. *Folk Medicine: A Vermont Doctor's Guide to Good Health.* New York: Holt, Rinehart and Winston, 1958.

Lasagna, L., et al. "A Study of the Placebo Response." *American Journal of Medicine* 16 (1954), p. 770.

Restak, R. "The Bronin Makes Its Own Narcotics." *Saturday Review,* March 5, 1977, pp. 7–11.

Sharpless, S. K. and J. Jaffe. "The Electrical Excitability of Isolated Cortex During Barbiturate Withdrawal." *Journal of Pharmacology and Experimental Therapy* 151 (1966), p. 321.

CHAPTER 6

Bunker, J. P. "Surgical Manpower: A Comparison of Operations in the United States and in England and Wales." *New England Journal of Medicine* 282 (1970), p. 135.

———. *The Anesthesiologist and the Surgeon: Partners in the Operating Room.* Boston: Little, Brown & Co., 1972.

Burch, G. E. and T. D. Giles. *Controversy in Surgery.* Edited by R. L. Varco and J. P. Delaney. Philadelphia: W. B. Saunders Co., 1976.

Lewis, C. E. "Variations in the Incidence of Surgery." *New England Journal of Medicine* 281 (1969), p. 880.

Loeser, J. D. "Dorsal Rhizotomy: Indications and Results." In *Advances in Neurology,* vol. 4, pp. 615–19. New York: Raven Press, 1974.

McCarthy, E. C. and C. Wedmer. "Effects of Screening by Consultants on Recommended Elective Surgical Procedures." *New England Journal of Medicine* 291 (1974), p. 25.

Mixer, W. J. and J. S. Barr. "Rupture of the Intervertebral Disc with Involvement of the Spinal Cord." *New England Journal of Medicine* 211 (1934), p. 210.

White, A. W. M. "Low-Back Pain in Men Receiving Workmen's Compensation." *Canadian Medical Association Journal* 101 (1969), p. 26.

CHAPTER 7

Black, R. G. and C. R. Chapman. "The SAD Index for Clinical Assessment of Pain." *Advances in Pain Research and Therapy,* vol. 1. Edited by J. J. Bonica and D. Albe-Fessard. New York: Raven Press, 1976.

Brena, S. F. and D. L. Koch. "A 'Pain Estimate Model' for Quantification and Classification of Chronic Pain States." *Anesthesiology Review* 2 (1975), pp. 8–13.

———. "Reliability of the 'Pain Estimate Model.'" *Anesthesiology Review* 4 (1976) pp. 28–29.

Chyatte, S., et al. "Chronic Pain States: How They Relate to Disability." *Proceedings of the Annual Meeting of the American Congress of Rehabilitation Medicine,* 1977.

Melzack, R. and W. S. Torgerson. "The Language of Pain." *Anesthesiology* 34 (1971), p. 50

Sternbach, R. A., et al. "Measuring the Severity of Clinical Pain." *Advances in Neurology,* vol. 4. New York: Raven Press, 1974.

CHAPTER 8

Halstead, L. S. and M. G. Halstead. "Chronic Illness and Humanism: Rehabilitation as a Model for Teaching Humanistic and Scientific Health Care." *Archives of Physical Medicine and Rehabilitation* 59 (1978), pp. 53–57.

Keele, K. D. *Anatomies of Pain.* Springfield, Ill.: C. C Thomas, 1957.

Sigerist, H. A. *A History of Medicine.* Oxford: Oxford University Press, 1951.

White, J. C. and W. H. Sweet. *Pain: Its Mechanisms and Neurosurgical Control.* Springfield, Ill.: C. C Thomas, 1955.

———. *Pain and the Neurosurgeon: A Forty-Year Experience.* Springfield, Ill.: C. C Thomas, 1969.

Zborowski, J. *People in Pain.* San Francisco: Jossey-Bass, 1969.

CHAPTER 9

Engel, G. L. and F. Reichmann. "Spontaneous and Experimentally Induced Depressions in an Infant with Gastric Fistula." *Journal of the American Psychoanalytic Association* 4 (1956), pp. 428–52.

Engel, G. L. "Psychogenic Pain and the Pain-Prone Patient." *American Journal of Medicine* 26 (1959), p. 899.

———. "Guilt, Pain and Success." *Psychosomatic Medicine* 24 (1962), p. 37.

Merskey, H. "Psychiatry Aspects of the Control of Pain." In *Advances in Pain Research and Therapy,* vol. 1. Edited by J. J. Bonica and D. Albe-Fessard. New York: Raven Press, 1976.

CHAPTER 10

Basmajian, J. V. "Control and Training of Individual Motor Units." *Science* 141 (1963), p. 440.

Bonica, J. J. *The Management of Pain.* Philadelphia: Lea & Febiger, 1953.

Fordyce, W. E., et al. "An Application of Behavior Modification Technique to a Problem of Chronic Pain." *Behavior Research and Therapy* 6 (1968), p. 105.

Mitchell, S. W. *Injuries of Nerves and Their Consequences.* J. B. Lippincott, 1874. Reprint. New York: Dover, 1965.

Morse, R. Personal Communication.

Peters, N., et al. *New England Rehabilitation Hospital Pain Unit Evaluation.* Interim Report. Unpublished data presented to the Annual Convention of the American Congress of Rehabilitation Medicine, 1976.

Shealy, C. N., et al. "Electrical Inhibition of Pain by Stimulation of the Dorsal Column: Preliminary Report." *Anesthesia-Analgesia* 46 (1967), p. 489.

CHAPTER 11

Brena, S. F. "Les Cliniques de la Douleur." *Anesthesiologie Européenne* 2 (1961), pp. 230–256.

Grossman, H. I. "Statement to the Subcommittee on Social Secu-*cial Security Proposals.* U. S. Government Printing Office, 1977.

Leff, D. N. "Management of Chronic Pain: Medicine, New Growth Industry." *Medical World News,* October 18, 1976, pp. 54–77.

CHAPTER 12

Brena, S. F. *Yoga and Medicine.* New York: Penguin, 1973.
Knowles, J. H. "The Responsibility of the Individual." *Daedalus,* Winter, 1977.

CHAPTER 13

Crue, B. L., et al. "Neurophysiology of Pain: Peripheral Aspects." *Bulletin of Los Angeles Neurological Sciences* 41 (1976).
Crue, B. L., ed. *Pain: Research and Treatment.* New York: Academic Press, 1975.
Eccles, J. C. "The Physiology of Imagination." In *Altered States of Awareness,* a special issue of *Scientific American,* 1972.
Melzack, R. and P. D. Wall. "Pain Mechanisms: A New Theory." *Science* 150 (1965), p. 971.

CHAPTER 14

DiCara, L. V. "Learning in the Autonomic Nervous System." *Scientific American* 222 (1970), p. 30.
Engel, B. T. "Operant Conditioning of Cardiac Function: A Status Report." *Psychophysiology* 9 (1972), pp. 161–77.
Wenger, M. A., et al. "Experiments in India on 'Voluntary' Control of the Heart and the Pulse." *Circulation* 24 (1900), pp. 1319–25.

CHAPTER 15

Livingston, W. K. *Pain Mechanisms: A Physiologic Interpretation of Causalgia and Its Related States.* New York: Macmillan, 1944.

Shapiro, A. P., et al. *Psychosomatic Classics: Selected Papers from Psychosomatic Medicine, 1939–1958.* White Plains, N.Y.: S. Karger, 1972.

Simons, D. C. "Muscle Pain Syndromes." *American Journal of Physical Medicine* 54 (1975).

CHAPTER 16

Brena, S. F. and I. P. Unikel. "Nerve Blocks and Contingency Management." *Advances in Pain Research and Therapy,* vol. 1, pp. 707–710. Edited by J. J. Bonica and D. Albe-Fessard. New York: Raven Press, 1976.

Fordyce, W. E. "Treating Chronic Pain by Contingency Management." In *Advances in Neurology,* vol. 4, pp. 583–89. New York: Raven Press, 1974.

Haley, J. *Strategies of Psychotherapy.* New York: Grune and Stratton, 1963.

Ullmann, L. P. and L. Krasner. *A Psychological Approach to Abnormal Behavior.* Englewood Cliffs, N. J.: Prentice-Hall, 1969.

CHAPTER 17

Benson, H. *The Relaxation Response.* New York: W. Morrow, 1975.

Birk, L., ed. *Behavioral Medicine: The Clinical Uses of Biofeedback.* New York: Grune and Stratton, 1973.

Ingelfinger, F. J. Editorial in *The New England Journal of Medicine.* February 24, 1977.

Jacobson, E. *Progressive Relaxation: A Physiological Approach.* Philadelphia: J. B. Lippincott, 1964.

Kamiya, J., et al. *Biofeedback and Self-Control: An Aldine Reader on the Regulation of Bodily Processes and Consciousness.* Chicago: Aldine, 1971.

Luthe, W. and J. H. Schultz *Autogenic Therapy,* vol. 1–4. New York: Grune and Stratton, 1970.

Wallace, R. K. and Benson, H. "The Physiology of Meditation." *Scientific American* 226 (1972), p. 84.

CHAPTER 18

Bonica, J. J. *Clinical Applications of Diagnostic and Therapeutic Nerve Blocks.* Springfield, Ill.: C. C Thomas, 1959.

Brena, S. F. "Current Status of Regional Analgesia for Diagnosis and Therapy." In *Regional Anesthesia.* Edited by J. J. Bonica. Philadelphia: F. A. Davis, 1971.

Kerr, F. "A Central Inhibitory Balance Theory." *Mayo Clinic Proceedings—Pain* 50 (1975), pp. 685–90.

Shealy, C. N. and D. Maurer. "Transcutaneous Nerve Stimulation for Control of Pain." *Surgical and Neurology* 2 (1974), pp. 45–47.

CHAPTER 19

Friedman, A. P., ed. *Research and Clinical Studies in Headache.* Baltimore: Williams and Wilkins, 1967.

Malmo, R. B. "Emotions and Muscle Tension: The Story of Asane." *Psychology Today* 3 (1970), p. 64.

Ostfield, A. M. *Common Headache Syndromes: Biochemistry, Pathophysiology, Therapy.* Springfield, Ill.: C. C Thomas, 1962.

Pearce, J. *Migraine: Clinical Features, Mechanisms and Management.* Springfield, Ill.: C. C Thomas, 1969.

Sainsbury, P. and J. F. Gibson. "Symptoms of Anxiety and Tension and Accompanying Physiological Changes in the Muscular System." *Journal of Neurology, Neurosurgery and Psychiatry* 17 (1954), pp. 215–24.

Wolff, H. G. *Headache and Other Head Pain.* 2nd ed. Oxford: Oxford Zuniversity Press, 1963.

CHAPTER 20

Cailliet, R. *Low Back Pain Syndrome.* 8th Printing. Philadelphia: F. A. Davis, 1976.

Cyriax, J. H. "Lumbago: Mechanisms of Dural Pain." *Lancet* 2 (1955), p. 427.

Nachemson, A. L. "The Lumbar Spine: An Orthopedic Challenge." *Spine* 1 (1976), pp. 59–71.

Shealy, C. N. "The Role of the Spinal Facets in Back and Sciatic Pain." *Headache* 14 (1974), pp. 101–4.

CHAPTER 21

Benson, E. H. and D. C. Zavala. "Importance of the Costochondral Syndrome in Evaluation of Chest Pain." *Journal of the American Medical Association* 156 (1954), pp. 1244–46.
Cailliet, R. *Neck and Arm Pain.* 10th Printing. Philadelphia: F. A. Davis, 1976.
Davis, D. "Radicular Syndromes with Emphasis on Chest Pain, Simulating Coronary Disease." Chicago: Year Book Medical Publishers, 1957.
Heberdeen, W. *Commentaries on the History and Cure of Disease.* London: T. Payne Co., 1802.

CHAPTER 22

Bellivean, F. and L. Richter. *Understanding Human Sexual Inadequacy.* New York: Bantam Books, 1970.
Kaplan, H. S. *The New Sex Therapy: Active Treatment of Sexual Dysfunctions.* New York: Brunner/Mazel, 1974.

CHAPTER 23

Schacter, S. *Emotions, Obesity and Crime.* New York: Academic Press, 1971.
Shmale, A. and H. Iher. "The Psychological Setting of Uterine Cervical Cancer." *Annals of the New York Academy of Sciences* 125 (1966), pp. 807–13.

CHAPTER 24

Bonica, J. J. "Pain Associated with Cancer and Other Neoplastic Diseases." In *The Management of Pain.* Philadelphia: Lea and Febiger, 1973.

Kübler-Ross, E. *Questions and Answers on Death and Dying.* New York: Macmillan, 1969.

Vanderpool, H. V. "The Ethics of Terminal Care." *Journal of the American Medical Association* 239 (1978), p. 850.

CHAPTER 25

The Bible (King James Version): Genesis 2:7. Job 4:2-6. Ecclesiastes 2:24. Matthew 6:3, 25–34, 26:37–46. Luke 6:48–49, 22:44–46. Ephesians 4:18–23. II Thessalonians 3:8–12.

The Song Celestial or Bhagavad-Gita: Chapter 4, p. 25; Chapter 12, pp. 78–79. Translated from the Sanskrit by Sir E. Arnold. Boston: Routledge and Kegan Paul, 1964.

The Bible of Bibles: pp. 148, 163–76. F. L. Riley, ed. J. F. Rowny Press, 1957.

Bakan, D. *Disease, Pain and Sacrifice: Toward a Psychology of Suffering.* Boston: Beacon Press, 1971.

Brena, S. F. *Pain and Religion: A Psychological Study.* Springfield, Ill.; C. C Thomas, 1972.

Bucke, R. M. *Cosmic Consciousness.* Rev. ed. New York: Dutton, 1968.

Cheney, S. *Men Who Have Walked with God.* New York: Dell, 1974.

Fuchs, V. R. *Who Shall Live? Health, Economics and Social Choice.* New York: Basic Books, 1974.

Johnston, C. *The Yoga Sutras of Patanjali.* London: J. M. Watkins, 1964.

Lynch, J. J. *The Broken Heart.* New York: Basic Books, 1977.

Pattison, E. M., ed. *Clinical Psychiatry and Religion.* Boston: Little, Brown & Co., 1969.

Westberg, C. *Good Grief.* Chicago: University of Illinois, A. Lincoln Medical School, 1961.

Yogananda, P. *The Science of Religion.* Los Angeles: Self-Realization Fellowship, 1967.

———. *Man's Eternal Quest.* Edited by Jane Brush. Los Angeles: Self-Realization Fellowship, 1975.

Index